Cholera and Nation

SUNY series, Studies in the Long Nineteenth Century

Pamela K. Gilbert, editor

Cholera and Nation

*Doctoring the Social Body
in Victorian England*

Pamela K. Gilbert

STATE UNIVERSITY OF NEW YORK PRESS

Cover: John Leech, "A Court for King Cholera," *Punch* Jul.–Dec. 1852. Courtesy of Lee Jackson, www.victorianlondon.org.

Published by
State University of New York Press, Albany

For information, contact State University of New York Press, Albany, NY
www.sunypress.edu

Production by Marilyn P. Semerad
Marketing by Anne M. Valentine

Library of Congress Cataloging-in-Publication Data

Gilbert, Pamela K.
    Cholera and nation : doctoring the social body in Victorian England /
Pamela K. Gilbert.
        p. cm. — (SUNY series, studies in the long nineteenth century)
    Includes bibliographical references and index.
    ISBN 978-0-7914-7343-6 (hardcover : alk. paper)
    ISBN 978-0-7914-7344-3 (pbk. : alk. paper)
    1. Cholera—England—History. 2. Cholera—Social aspects—England—History.
    3. Cholera—England—Religious aspects—Christianity. I. Title. II. Series.
        [DNLM: 1. Cholera—history—England. 2. Attitude to Health—England.
    3. History, 19th Century—England. 4. Politics—England. 5. Public Health
    Practice—history—England. 6. Religion and Medicine—England. WC 262
    G465c 2008]

RA644.C3.G55 2008
616.9'32—dc22
                                                                    2007014883

10 9 8 7 6 5 4 3 2 1

CONTENTS

ACKNOWLEDGMENTS

AS IS USUAL WITH ANY PROJECT, I owe thanks to too many people to count. Institutions first: I must mention the generous assistance and friendly atmosphere of the Wellcome Institute for the History of Medicine, and especially Sally Bragg, who makes it all function smoothly. Thanks too to the Wellcome Library, and most especially Lesley Hall. The British Library, where I have consumed many books and more tea, has made this book possible. Finally, the PRO, the London Guildhall, the archivists at St. Bart's, the Royal College of Physicians, and the East London Hospital, and the interlibrary loan staff at the University of Florida all contributed to this project, as did material support from the University of Florida and the NEH.

Of my colleagues, all of whom are important sources of stimulation and support, I would like to especially thank fellow-Victorianist Chris Snodgrass. My other colleagues and friends Don Ault, Marsha Bryant, Kim Emery, Susan Hegeman, Phil Wegner, Stephanie Smith, John Murchek, Sid Dobrin, Terry Harpold, Judy Page, Apollo Amoko, Leah Rosenberg, John Van Hook, Pat Craddock, and Brandon Kershner have given me invaluable intellectual, social, and emotional nourishment. Special thanks to Malini Schueller, who has read with me and helped me clarify my thinking. Thanks always to Kenneth Kidd, who read and commented on the manuscript, and for his unfailing enthusiasm and sense of fun, and to Tace Hedrick whose friendship and conversation, scholarly and otherwise, sustain me. I must express my gratitude also to Chair John Leavey, whose support has been important to this project, as has his outstanding leadership in the department during a most difficult time. Of colleagues outside of Florida, I must thank particularly Michael Levenson, Elizabeth Langland, and Jim Kincaid. Of many correspondents, Talia Shaffer has been a particularly wonderful interlocutor, as have Nancy Armstrong, Tim Alborn, Lesley Hall (over and above her help as a librarian and archivist), Steve Sturdy, Ryan Johnson, Susan Zieger, Yopie Prins, David Wayne Thomas, Martha Vicinus, Mark Harrison, Peter Logan, Gustavo Verdesio, and many others whose comments have at one time or another been crucial to my thinking about the larger cholera project. Many graduate students have contributed to my thinking and have helped make my intellectual environment a productive one, and I'd like to thank them all but must single out Heather Milton and Madhura Bandyopadyay. Clare Ford Wille and Peter Shahbenderian have shared their home with me and supported me, this book, and the larger cholera project unreservedly for the seemingly endless series of summer research visits it has taken to see it completed. Long phone conversations with Meryl Strichartz and Nicolet de Rose reminded me there was a world outside my office and people I loved within it. I need especially to thank some of my readers for the State University of New York Press, and at the press itself, James Peltz, a superb acquisitions editor, and Charles Shepherdson, on the press's editorial board, whose perceptive and supportive commentary, produced when he was on leave and might well have preferred to do other things, made an enormous difference to this book. This work or work related to it has been presented at a number of conferences and working groups, where many scholars have influenced my thinking. These include the Modern Language Association, various Society for the Social History of Medicine and Wellcome conferences, the North American Conference of British Studies, and the Victorians' Institute. And who can begin to calculate what is owed by all of us to the collective wisdom and goodwill of the VICTORIA list and the indefatigable Patrick Leary? To all of you who daily prove that the whole is more than the sum of its parts, my heartfelt thanks.

Portions of material on pages 17–21, 30–35, 38–39, 43–44, and 47–53 first appeared in an article entitled "'A Sinful and Suffering Nation': Cholera and the Evolution of Medical and Religious Authority in Britain, 1832–1866," published in *Nineteenth Century Prose*, 25.1 (Spring 1998): 35–59, and reappear here with their gracious permission.

INTRODUCTION

Human knowledgeability [*sic*] is always bounded. The flow of action continually produces consequences which are unintended by actors, and these unintended consequences also may form unacknowledged conditions of action in a feedback fashion. Human history is created by intentional activities, but is not an intended project; it persistently eludes efforts to bring it under conscious direction. However, such attempts are continually made by human beings, who operate under the threat and the promise of the circumstance that they are the only creatures who "make" their history in cognizance of that fact.
—Anthony Giddens, *The Constitution of Society*

It is no fable . . . sin is the very root and cause of cholera. We never would have found it in this land had there not been some flagrant guilt to punish . . . there is some alarming increase to our national guilt . . . it is our duty, with the Spirit's aid, to search it out. Oh for skill to find it!
    —Reverend D. F. Jarman, "The Cholera, Its True Cause"

The Cholera comes—Rejoice! Rejoice!
He shall be lord of the swarming town!
And mow them down, and mow them down!
        —Charles Mackay, "The Mowers—
        An Anticipation of the Cholera, 1848"

BETWEEN 1832 AND 1866, four cholera epidemics devastated Britain. In his 1846 introduction to the sixth edition of his popular medical text, George Gregory styles cholera "the most malignant of the many maladies to which mankind is obnoxious" (vi). Medical accounts of cholera in 1832 usually

1

opened, not with reference to typhoid or small pox, but to the Great Plague.[1] Certainly British Victorians made it the subject of a vastly disproportionate fear and interest, perhaps because of its foreignness and the speed and drama with which it killed. Cholera is a waterborne disease caused by a comma-shaped bacillus, or vibrio, which is generally transmitted between humans via the fecal-oral route. It enters the human body through ingestion of contaminated water or food, and multiplies in the gut. Untreated, it kills about fifty percent of those infected quickly—usually within a few days—through rapid dehydration.[2]

Because dehydration was so rapid, nineteenth-century patients went from apparent health to a state of shrunken weakness very quickly—skin loose and shrivelled, lips drawn back from the teeth, eye sockets collapsed. Circulatory collapse due to low blood pressure also caused cyanosis (blue complexion) especially at the extremities. Muscles spasmed painfully and violently, causing patients to scream and thrash helplessly until exhausted and weak. The next state, collapse, was marked by stupor. Although patients were conscious, they tended to be unresponsive and unable to vocalize, except in a whistling whisper—the infamous *vox cholerae* or choleric voice. Soon after, these hardly recognizable patients—pinched, blue-black, and contorted—died.

In 1866, physician Edward Goodeve identifies the first stages of cholera: invasion, development, collapse, and reaction. After reaction, the feverish "second stage" might set in.[3] In this stage the less than fifty percent who survived the first stage might fall victim to what Victorians called "consecutive fever," resembling typhus—probably a result of opportunistic infection. Although this stage was not as dangerous, still many died of or were permanently damaged by it. Occasional mention is made of gangrene resulting from prolonged collapse or other irritation of sensitive tissue resulting in permanent damage, for example, sloughing of the cornea. Altogether, it was a terrifying and piteous spectacle, leaving medics and relatives little time to react rationally.[4]

Fluid loss occurred primarily through copious, constant, and uncontrollable diarrhea, and to a lesser extent vomiting. The diarrhea consisted, after a brief initial period, not of fecal matter, but of the characteristic "rice water" evacuations—a watery discharge with rice husk like particles, which were actually the serous or watery content of the blood and bits of the epithelial lining of the intestine that began to slough off as the discharges were prolonged. Bedding and clothing were unavoidably soaked with these clear evacuations. It is easy to see how, even without poor sewerage, contamination of utensils, food, and drinking water would take place in a small dwelling, especially when caregivers neither knew they should nor were consistently able to clean their hands. Further, poor sewerage did cause contamination to drinking water supplies, and in the warmer months, water was often drunk cold. Even in cold weather, beer might be adulterated with unboiled water, and many who were very poor could not waste fuel on thoroughly boiling water for tea or cooking, had they even known they should do so.

Just being poor was, and is, likely to result in a generally debilitated state of health that made one more liable to infection: doctors now believe that a healthy stomach's highly acid environment usually kills a moderate cholera inoculum before it can reach the bowel. The other major variable in determining the exposure to infection ratio is size of the inoculum: that is, the more vibrios go into one's body, the more likely it is that the disease will be contracted and be proportionately severe. But until later in the nineteenth century, cholera was widely thought to be caused by miasma or an "epidemic constitution" of the air and weather, perhaps exacerbated by decomposing wastes and their smell. Richard Evans has pointed out, "Cholera broke through the precarious barriers erected against physicality in the name of civilization . . . the thought that one might be seized with an uncontrollable, massive attack of diarrhoea . . . in the presence of scores or hundreds of respectable people, must have been almost as terrifying as the thought of death itself" (*Death in Hamburg* 229).

Cholera's entry into Britain late in 1831 has been extensively documented.[5] Quarantine was briefly tried, but quickly yielded to merchants' outrage and the apparent failure of quarantine in Eastern Europe. As historian Michael Durey points out, though, those months, the hottest of the year, might have been decisive in retarding cholera's progress until cooler weather would help minimize mortality (26); that is, if victims died too quickly, there was less chance of their traveling to infect new areas. Regardless, it finally entered Britain in Sunderland and then quickly spread, causing the worst London mortality in 1832. It was perceived immediately as an urban disease, despite the fact that death rates were comparatively higher in small villages (Morris 38–41). It returned in 1848–1849 to exact a much more devastating toll, and then again in 1854–1855 and 1866–1867. After that, although it raged again on the continent in the 1870s and early '90s, it did not cross over the channel in sufficient force to rate as an epidemic. Previous to what came to be called "the 1832 epidemic" in Britain, one pandemic began in India in 1817 that did extend through Europe but did not cross the channel.[6] Epidemiologist Dhiman Barua argues that there were earlier epidemics of cholera outside of India, and cites an impressive array of descriptions to support that conclusion; however, as Barua points out, confusing terminology and vague descriptions make it difficult to be sure what disease is being described, and many historians believe that 1817 was the first world pandemic. Regardless, in the 1830s, most British medics believed it was a new disease, and found it quite recalcitrant, whether a foreign disease or a new form of "English cholera" or autumnal diarrhea.

This terrifying illness entered England in a period of intense social and political change: reform of the political process and of voting, changes in the role of the state church, and the threat (some thought) of revolution: in short, it was a moment in which the relation of the state to the population was being substantially reconfigured. Over the course of the four cholera outbreaks, rampant fear in the population about an unknown and lethal disease prompted responses by the clergy as well as government officials, and a new class of medical authorities emerged. These groups wrestled for control of authority to define the meanings of the epidemics, as social space was changing, the definition of the nation was being hammered out in relation to class politics, and legal reforms were being hotly contested.

This book began as a study of the social body in its relationship to the cholera epidemics of 1832–1867, a topic in which I had become interested during my earlier work in discourses of disease and the social body in relation to popular novels. I quickly discovered that the rhetoric of the sanitary movement and the impact of medical science—prompted in some respects by those epidemics and often brought into public discourse in relation to them—permeates the entire culture and is inseparable from the larger political and cultural history of the nation. My study then split into multiple book projects. This volume focuses on the reception and rhetorical uses of the cholera epidemics that swept England four times from the early 1830s to the mid-1860s. Discussions of the cholera made definitions of the body and its health central to imaginings of nation and representation during the first Reform Bill debates that coincided with the earliest epidemic. These rhetorical uses of the body persisted as liberal government staked its claims to authority on the management of the social body through the medical question of public health.[7] The centrality of the body and its health to England's (and Britain's) sense of itself as a modern nation made in turn for an easy movement toward racialized and gendered ideals of the nation at mid-century that would form the basis of early twentieth-century notions of nationalism.

As both Benedict Anderson and Eric Hobsbawm have argued, national identity is based on stories citizens tell themselves. In nineteenth-century Britain, these tales attached other stories—chief among them, the stories of public health, the rise of liberal government, the justification of the Empire— to the trope of the body and the narrative of its healthy evolution. From Walter Scott's novels to Young Englandism to the revival of Arthurian legends later in the century, Britons used the legends of antiquity to legitimate their own identity in a national narrative that reached back over "empty time" and the idea of a wholly modern scientific progress as fundamental to a national narrative. This story emphasized both essential, immutable characteristics based on racial and geographic heritage and a teleology of national self-actualization and improvement through knowledge gathering and technological implementation of the policies implied by that knowledge. The knowledge deemed most valuable in this period privileged the observation and measurement of what were perceived as objective, material phenomena—bodies, geography—and recreated government as their management. The professionals who designed, managed, and were the instruments of these processes authorized themselves as speakers for the nation and therapeutic managers of the nation's social body. The notion of the social body itself became a way to talk about the connection between the public sphere of nation and the private sphere of individuals, while citizenship—both as a way of defining the person as a member of the national social body and as the institutional link between nation and state—became the measure of its health.

The social body, as elaborated by Michel Foucault, Mary Poovey, and others, refers to the metaphorical description of the population as a unified and specifically corporeal whole. Although this concept had a long history in the early modern period, it took on a particular importance in the late eighteenth and early nineteenth centuries, as discussions of the social body coincided with a new view of the role of the state as manager of physical health and facilitator of social cohesion. With the advent of new statistical practices to measure the population, recasting it within a grid of closely related knowledge gathering and management practices, the social body came to be understood increasingly as a mass of standardized and deviant bodies, making up a whole whose health was dependent on the essential equivalence of its parts.

This notion of equivalent bodies was related to a concept of fundamentally equivalent subjectivities, which emerged most clearly in late eighteenth- and nineteenth-century liberalism. This equivalence was not social equality but the equivalence of an innate self, prior to culture, that was "naturally" similar across classes and that naturally manifested certain desires (for shelter, financial security, cleanliness, etc.). If the subject did not manifest those natural desires, ill health—moral, economic, and political—would be the result. Poverty and vice, then, were reconfigured as less the result of a fallen nature than of the perversion of human nature through unnatural circumstances, such as living in the conditions contingent upon urban poverty. Moral health came to be seen as contingent upon, as well as coterminous with, physical health.

The advent of epidemic disease in urban areas lent both focus and urgency to this understanding of the social body, as well as providing it with a vocabulary based in the notion of a physically healthy body as the basis of the modern state. These narratives of national identity to which nineteenth-century writers appealed were hardly coherent; indeed, they were fragmentary and often self-contradictory. But some common themes emerged out the welter of general discourse: the nation is a body that can suffer ills; the political class and the elite professions have some standing to speak for and to the ills of that body; the larger populace is one of virtuous poor/workers who have special roles both as mute representatives of Englishness—the body for which the elites speak—and as a potential threat, whose massed mindless energy may be directed destructively against the social body as a whole; and disease enters the national body through such weak links as paupers, foreigners, and the inappropriately feminine.

Although there are problems with such an all-encompassing definition of nationalism as Katherine Verdery's—"the political utilization of the symbol nation through discourse and political activity, as well as the sentiment that draws people into responding to this symbol's use" ("Whither 'Nation' and 'Nationalism'?" 227)—this generalized discursive mobilization of "nation" as a significant term is a precondition of nationalism, as well as one of its modes of operation. Patrick Brantlinger observes that studies of nationalism tend to address its explicit military and political manifestations "while failing to grapple with the easy, everyday, or unconscious operation of nationality as a powerful factor in individual identity formation" (*Fictions of State* 4). It is this everyday "utilization" with which I most closely concern myself. As Verdery notes, studying "nation" as a symbol involves seeing it as multivalent and taking its meanings in large part within the conflicts that seek to mobilize its power ("Whither 'Nation'" 230). Linda Colley's landmark study, *Britons*, makes clear that nation was consolidated in Britain as an overarching identity within which other identities (local, ethnic) were not necessarily effaced, but were co-opted in complicated ways. However, as she also shows, nation still requires an "us" and a "them" system of identifications, and in the 1830s, much of that system revolved around Protestantism. What emerges over and over in the documents I discuss is that, by 1832, nation was already available—and preeminent—as a symbol available for unity, power, and authority. It was often used, however, to impeach the authority of some interlocutor, whose power to speak for any kind of unity, let alone a national one, was in question. If the nation-state was, as Brantlinger has argued, created through a process "whereby debt, absence, and powerlessness are transubstantiated, mainly through class exploitation at home and war abroad, into their opposites—wealth, a plenitude of laws and institutions, and power" (*Fictions* 20), then nation as a concept was mobilized discursively over the mid-century not only to unify oppositions, but, through precisely the medium of anxiety about those fissures, to neurotically insist upon the reality of that unity, and the imperviousness of the position that claimed it to critique.

The development of liberal government required unifying narratives, such as nation. And, as Foucault argued, it required the rise of a professional class, and techniques of governance based on the legitimating force of scientific knowledge, to administer the great unities upon which the state's progress depended. Medicine and law both assumed unprecedented importance in this period, but medicine particularly changed in status as it moved into the position of a kind of secular established clergy, preempting the clergy's place as interpreter of events affecting the social body. Medicine evolved toward acceptance as a public, elite profession, while simultaneously an ideal of bourgeois professional leadership emerged. At the same time, science became an ever more important component of Britain's vision of itself as a modern nation, and the Empire self-consciously styled itself as a ruler through archival knowledge.[8]

As Foucault has argued, the move toward modern liberal government was marked by "governmentalities"—the development of bodies of knowledge that are also practices—particularly in regard to biopolitics (the management of populations) through public health, mortality returns, the census, and the like. These data enabled governments both to know about the movements and living habits of their subjects and also to mobilize consent among those subjects to governmental aims, rather than relying on brute power. The discourses and practices that emerged in Britain in regard to these developments authorized themselves with the rhetoric of national identity, interest, and improvement. In this volume, I engage those associated with the development of the medical profession and the sanitary movement (related but not identical categories) and its relation to the emerging concept of the social body.

What would come to be understood over the course of the period as "public health"—especially in relationship to epidemic disease and sanitary issues—had a privileged role in the discourses of the social body. As historian of medicine Charles Rosenberg has noted,

> An epidemic has a dramaturgic form . . . [it] takes on the quality of a pageant—mobilizing communities to act out propitiatory rituals that incorporate and reaffirm fundamental social values and modes of understanding. It is their public character and dramatic intensity—along with unity of time and place—that make epidemics as well suited to the concerns of moralists as well as to the research of scholars seeking an understanding of the relationship among ideology, social structure and the construction of particular selves. (*Explaining Epidemics* 279)

Mary Poovey has read Victorian medic James Kay-Shuttleworth's use of cholera as a master metaphor for all the social body's ills and justification for middle-class rule of society in contradistinction to class-based legislation (*Making a Social Body*), and I would extend her observations to note that this use of cholera was commonplace in this period, even as it was also used to challenge such values. Public health emerged in this period as a domain of knowledge and intervention as a result of the tendency toward governmentalization; the opportunity arose in response to (particularly urban) epidemics, and cholera has generally been accorded the role of prime actor in this drama. Although some historians have reacted against what they see as its undue prominence in historiography (R. J. Morris went so far as to claim that the impact that cholera actually had on legislation was negligible), I agree with

Richard Evans that cholera had a very important impact, which is missed if one looks only for direct causal relationships in the narrowest sense ("Epidemics and Revolutions").[9] Those historians who, like Morris or Michael Durey, measured cholera only in terms of its threat to the "stability of society," are almost bound to find that it had little direct impact, especially in that there is no clear definition of what such stability would consist of.

It is important to remember, of course, that the cholera itself did not *cause* the public health movement. Had the conditions not been right for acceptance, however grudging, of public health as the business of government, and had the beginnings of statistical knowledge not made public health as a knowledge project feasible, cholera alone would have done little. But the conditions *were* right, and the dramatic eruption of an alien and frightening epidemic during conditions of Reform agitation provided unique practical and narrative opportunities, despite the fact that cholera was hardly as important a threat as the routine depredations of diseases already endemic to the Isles, like typhus and typhoid. Such diseases, of course, also played an important part in prompting sanitary reform, but cholera focused public fear and resolve in a way no endemic illness could.

Although I am not principally interested in the "dramaturgical" form identified by Rosenberg, I am concerned with narrative forms of knowledge. Medics used the public attention elicited by the epidemics and responses to them to create a public platform for the profession; they mobilized discourses of nation and the social to add force to their position, and in so doing, contributed to the formation of those discourses themselves. Just as epidemic disease became a privileged symbol for threats to the social body, cholera became the most dramatic icon of all such visitations. For these reasons, public health and the cholera epidemics provide an especially fruitful source of stories about the social body and the "condition of England."

The body itself is a key signifier. Basic representative of a materiality that is malleable yet limited, the body came to function, in this period, as both the index and the metaphor of the nation. Individual bodies and their ills, as representatives of classes and populations, became indexes of the condition of that less tangible entity, the social body. Early on, the social itself, in both its physical and moral manifestations, came to be understood as a medicalized physical entity that could be fixed, observed, and dissected, both through the individual bodies of its subjects and in toto (or en masse), in the form of statistics. The key locus of this body's construction was in public medicine, a combination of medical views of the body and specific sanitary formulations that enabled medics to speak from the position of a public profession. Medical theory and research contributed to a changing view of the body popularized and taken up publicly in specific ways that related to the larger social project of the mid-nineteenth century.

In the first part of this book, I show how the coming of the cholera, and the early public health movement associated with it, reacted with the unrest of the Reform era to create specific opportunities for various interest groups to rhetorically position themselves in relation to the nation and the social body. Each of these groups claimed to "read" a different relationship between the individual and the larger national community: clergy, medics, sanitarians, and labor radicals all seized the opportunity to interpret the early cholera epidemics, laying the groundwork for future discussions. Chapter 1 explores the politico-religious response to the first epidemic in 1832 that set the terms of the debate for subsequent responses. Chapter 2 traces these debates during the following epidemics, as sanitary and medical responses to this early discourse emerge. Medics began during this time to make efforts to gain credibility as public interpreters of the social body and its health. Chapter 3 surveys the responses of the poor and of political radicals throughout the period. These groups were largely placed in the position of reacting to and appropriating dominant discourses; yet, their writings and actions also display an adept manipulation of the debate to specific political and practical ends. Each group attempted to claim authority to assign meaning to the epidemics, and each posited their response in terms of the nation and its political and moral health.

The second part turns from the larger public sphere to the explicitly medical construction of the body and its relation to understandings of public health. Developing understandings of the body depended on increasing professionalization and a shift to a surgical and histological model of the body, away from the old systemic vision of the elite class of medics, the physicians. Chapter 4 explores the development of medicine from an amorphous group of practitioners to a profession defined by the perpetuation of elite knowledges (or *savoirs* in Foucault's terms) and specialization. This process of building credibility for medicine as a profession was closely related to medicine's ability to claim a position of authority in the public sphere, and the presence of epidemic disease enabled medics to claim a role in making public policy, prescribing for populations rather than individuals. This new authority allowed medics to situate moral and social prescriptions in a discourse on health and hygiene. Chapter 5 traces the ways in which increasing specialization and the advent of new medical models also allowed for a shift in the view of the body from one that privileged a balanced intake and excretion in order to maintain homeostasis to one that emphasized the essential dangerousness of any material entering or exiting the body—indeed, one that insisted on the essentially dangerous nature of the body itself. As medics became speakers for and ministers to the national body, medicine began to foreground questions of race and gender, and nation became identified not only with the healthy body, but a specifically Northern European, masculine body. Chapter 6 examines the racial and gendered aspects of cholera in medical discourse and their relation to an emerging vision of the nation as consisting of paradigmatic white and masculine bodies threatened by encroaching colonial blackness and feminization.

If political and religious discourses surrounding cholera shaped the early medical response to the disease, the transformation of the medical position into one of public oversight meant that medical discourse had in turn a strong impact on writing for the general public. Part 3 turns again to the public sphere, tracing the elaboration of these connections in the realm of literary production. As was true in political and religious discussion, representations of cholera in literature tended to be closely identified with the state of the social body, and medical management of cholera with state management of social ills. Chapter 7 surveys the appearance of cholera in several literary contexts, from poetry to didactic novels aimed at the poor to George Eliot's use of disease in *Middlemarch* and *Felix Holt*. Charles Kingsley—Anglican minister, sanitarian, and novelist—provides an excellent, and hitherto neglected, case study, and chapter 8 provides a detailed reading of his work. His ouevre is a particularly strong example of the confluence of racial, gendered, medical, national, and religious discourses in the novel, the privileged form for the elaboration of narratives of bourgeois individual development. Following Carlyle and Arnold, Kingsley concerned himself with devising a gendered national narrative constructed around notions of racial identity, both as a novelist and historian.

Scholars have often shied away from much analysis of Kingsley's racial theories, in part because such ideas are offensive to us now, but also because Kingsley's ideas resist analysis, seeming chaotic and self-contradictory, as his culture's and his own understanding of race and racial politics fluctuated over the course of his career. His confusion about race—and determination to grapple with it—reflect a central problem of liberal Britain; how could an inclusive social body based on a notion of fundamental human equality be made to mesh with nineteenth-century understandings of Caucasian and specifically English superiority? What was the relationship of that national social body to imperial expansion? His "cholera novel," *Two Years Ago*, provides a case study of how these connections were elaborated within the paradigm of public health and gestures more broadly toward the stakes of definitions of nationhood based on bodies.

This volume examines much previously overlooked material—sermons, medical textbooks, and the like—and elaborates a historical and rhetorical relationship between nation, cholera, and the body that has not previously been discussed. That said, the epidemics themselves are a well-worn topic, and I offer here no new discoveries in epidemiological history per se. However, this study does attempt a modest reconceptualization of the possibilities for "doing" medical history, for how it may be approached. First, it places medical history in this period right where it belongs—at the center of cultural formation and political discourse. Second, it moves away from the intensive study of individuals, scientific discoveries, and legislative policies common in the frequently teleological model of current medical history toward the examination of medical discourses circulating throughout the culture, attempting a partial construction of a certain moment's "field of vision." The average reader of newspapers—and even the average medic—was probably far less interested in the specifics of which individual doctors were working with sanitary reformer Edwin Chadwick than in trying to make some sense of the disease out of the information being disseminated by those who could claim expert authority. While the detailed study of specific individuals in key positions is crucial to an understanding of the development of specific policies, there is also something to be gained from having a sense of the discursive climate to which they contributed and in which they acted. (It is this conviction that has also influenced my choice to include frequent, detailed excerpts from primary documents, most of which are not readily available to readers.)

I have depended heavily on the work of Michel Foucault and Mary Poovey. First, I have used some of Foucault's insights in the history of medicine and government, but more importantly, I consider my project to be genealogical in his sense of the term. That is, this study involves the analysis of knowledge structures that undergird and create the conditions of possibility for both knowledge categories (for example, medicine) and for social relations. Poovey's analysis of the making of the social body is fundamental for me, and I see my work here as depending upon and extending her analysis of the category of the social. This project also aims to restore a sense of the importance of political discourse to the history of "power/knowledge." Foucault has concentrated on showing the importance of large shifts in the construction of power and knowledge, and I show here how various groups attempted to access these new sources of authority. However, these human actions may, in turn, change the terrain of power and knowledge in ways that are not determined by epistemological (or genealogical) change per se.

In *The Order of Things*, Foucault identifies a shift in underlying knowledge structures that initiated what he calls the modern period as taking place around 1800 (*Order* xxii). This change allowed for the invention of, among other things, humanity (*Order* 386). It certainly made possible the modern organization of the human sciences. In this shift, the basis of knowledge changed to a classification and understanding of an "internal principle" that was "alien to the domain of the visible" (*Order* 227). This change, which made possible the work of both Thomas Malthus and David Ricardo and structurally aligned their concerns, emphasized the finitude of human life and productive energy (*Order* 259). It is this focus which also allows, in Foucault's analysis, for the move, in Georges Cuvier's work from the focus on the organ as a visible structure to the focus on invisible function (*Order* 264). Human life as productivity is defined by death, the exhaustion of resources. This new understanding is reflected in tissue theory, which posits death as a principle internal to life. And this understanding also valorizes the medic as the social manager par excellence. As Foucault went on to discuss in *The Birth of the Clinic*, the new way of classifying knowledge gave importance to epidemics as political problems in the management of populations (*Birth* 25). The transition to morbid anatomy and pathology privileged a medical gaze that could perceive what was not visible on the surface, or indeed, to the unskilled observer, the "visible invisible" (*Birth* 149). Disease in this period "breaks away from the metaphysics of evil," from "counter-nature," and takes its place as a force "embodied in the living body" (*Birth* 196). The body can be perceived as a unity and as continuous with the environment in a new way; the laws that govern economies can be aligned with the laws that govern population. I discuss how these transitions in the understanding of death as a management problem and toward scientific expertise as the basis of management ability enable medics to step into the public arena as the interlocutors of the clergy and of politicians.

This book relates to a number of other studies published in the last several years, both within and without the immediate domain of medical history and literature. Here I will name just a few that I have found particularly useful and that intersect with my project in interesting ways. Ian Hacking's foundational 1990 book, *The Taming of Chance*, traces the development of understanding of statistical laws and the move, in the West, from a deterministic model to one in which chance played a significant role over the period of the late eighteenth and nineteenth centuries. One effect of this complex and multiform adjustment was in the field of medicine, in which, Hacking argues, François-Joseph-Victor Broussais's work on pathology established that the laws of disease followed the same laws as those of the organism generally, being defined as excess, rather than being a state completely separate and apart from that of the healthy body. Related to this change, questions of the goodness or corruption of human nature were displaced by discussions of norms and normalcy (Hacking 160–61). A statistical concept of the norm became a value-laden aspirational goal: to be normal, or to foster normalcy. And indeed, as he observes, most of the statistics used for purposes of government derived from what were considered states or acts of deviancy: disease, suicide, prostitution (3). Catherine Gallagher's most recent book, *The Body Economic*, works to build a coherent and intriguing history of how the nineteenth-century development of moral philosophy and its daughter disciplines displaced questions of the transcendent meaning and worth of human life from the spiritual to the organic—life and bodily pleasures. These areas of knowledge underlay not only the disciplines of economics, but of statecraft. She divides the two main foci of these new studies into the well-known Foucauldian term bioeconomics (the management of population, mortality, and so forth), and her own term, "somaeconomics," the "theorization of economic behavior in terms of the emotional and sensual feelings that are both causes and consequences of economic behavior" (3). As the new study of "economics" seemed to become increasingly concerned with the former, somaeconomics seemed to become more the domain of the "human" sciences. Gallagher aims to restore our understanding of early economics and, indeed, nineteenth-century thought more generally, as encompassing both these questions more simultaneously than we allow. The best studies of medicine and literature in the period examine them in their contexts as a continuity of discourses that are yet, of course, inflected and empowered by their contexts of origin, their "disciplinary precincts," as Lawrence Rothfield puts it in his powerful study of medicine and realist fiction in the nineteenth century, *Vital Signs*—a project not only archaeological (or genealogical) in the Foucauldian sense, but simply epistemological as well. Both Hacking and Gallagher are interested in the discursive matrixes out of which are produced the notion of normativity and its deep relations to the biological, which is my subject here. I aim here to show how medicine, more closely concerned with both of what Gallagher calls bio- and somaeconomics than perhaps many twentieth-century historians have realized, could move toward understanding and placing something as seemingly baldly physiological as cholera in a central relationship to questions of citizenship, morality, and the state, and also how medics could move toward a position of centrality in speaking to those questions. The identification of "norms" of health and the normative body with goodness as a goal of governing, and of the ideal body with the nation, signally changed the direction of discourses related to domains as apparently discrete as government, religion, medicine.

Because I do address the emerging role of medics as speakers for the nation, this work also intersects with recent debates on the nature of Victorian statecraft and theories of government. Although this project draws heavily on Foucault's work on the histories of knowledge and medicine, it is, as aforementioned, heavily informed in its approach to questions of power by his later work on governmentalities. Lauren Goodlad's wonderful *Victorian Literature and the Victorian State* works from this later Foucauldian perspective as well. She traces the debates about the formation of state and civil authorities that would be "pastoral" in nature, fostering correct forms of individuality. In this sense, her work dovetails with mine, as this volume provides a glimpse at the debate about a specific transition in secular pastoral authority, the forms of that authority, and the knowledge claims on which it was based. Amanda Anderson's *The Powers of Distance*, which examines the attraction to and anxiety about the notion of critical distance involved in Victorian notions of cosmopolitanism and citizenship, may seem less obviously connected to my project. However, the critical distance basic to the medical and scientific gaze, and medics' claims to authority in the public sphere based on that coolly rational distance, are intimately connected to the notions of the state and appropriate citizenship Anderson traces so ably. Within medical history specifically, Nadja Durbach's excellent *Bodily Matters*, on the history of the anti-vaccination movement in England from 1853–1907, uses her very different topic to accomplish some parallel aims to my study. As do Goodlad and I, she claims Foucault as her starting point, but, also as we do, she examines how various groups access power in the struggle for political and individual agency, rather than analyzing the disciplinary production of the consenting subject. She also focuses on the intersection between the body as the key contested site of power/knowledge, and its relation to the state and citizenship, as well as the intersection between expert knowledges, politics, and popular discourses. These diverse books are all part of a larger project of refocusing on agency after the perceived deterministic excesses of earlier Foucauldian scholarship on the Victorian period inspired by such work as *Discipline and Punish*. Like the work of political scholars such as Nikolas Rose, they focus less upon the state as a central actor than as one element within "various incarnations of what one might term 'the will to govern,' as it is enacted in a multitude of pro-grammes, strategies, tactics, devices . . . aimed at the conduct of the individu-als, groups, populations—and indeed oneself . . . in multiple circuits of power, connecting a diversity of authorities and forces, within a whole variety of com-plex assemblages" (Rose 5).

In tracing the representation, reception, and significance of cholera in this period, we can clearly see not only how cholera was "used" by various groups to advance their arguments and anchor understandings of identity, we can also see the powerful but aleatory relationship between cholera, the body, and nation. Had cholera not come, liberal govermentality would still have devel-oped and would still have been based in part on the management of popula-tion. But the entailments of that management might not have been rooted so aggressively in the healthy male body of the worker and threats to that body constructed as foreign invasion. Had the cholera epidemics not begun in the tense era of Reform debate, discussions of political representation and the "condition of England question" might also have been figured quite differ-ently, and eugenic theories might have become central to ideas of the nation's body later and in other forms. Cholera's ambiguous gift was the specific shape of an understanding of nation centrally grounded in the health of the body, a centrality that shaped Britain's understanding of itself throughout the nine-teenth century and beyond.

PART I

A Sinful and Suffering Nation

It is no fable . . . sin is the very root and cause of cholera.
—Reverend D. F. Jarman, "The Cholera, Its True Cause . . ."

. . . It is my opinion, as a man,
That trade as [*sic*] long been at a stand,
There's thousands starving through the land
And that's the Cholera Morbus.
—Broadsheet, "Cholera Morbus!"

1

A Sinful Nation

1832

MANY STUDIES HAVE ELABORATED the medical history of the epidemics and a few, like R. J. Morris's, trace some of the social impact. However, very little attention has been paid to the religious response or the epidemic's political uses in the franchise reform debates, related and very important aspects of the cholera's social and political impact on public debate for many years to come. This and the following two chapters examine how cholera was taken up by various interest groups and immediately discursively wedded to the other major public concern of the time: the debates surrounding the 1832 Reform Bill. The Reform Bill, hotly contested, aimed to expand the franchise to include some male members of the middle class and also to reform the electoral system, eliminating rotten boroughs and the bribing of electors. Coming on the heels of religious reform bills that increased tolerance of Catholics and dissenters and amid fears of revolution, the Reform Bill seemed to some to herald the dissolution of society and to others, the coming of a just and perfect state. The apparent volatility of society and its institutions was linked in the press to the mysterious threat of the new illness.

CHOLERA AND THE CHURCH IN 1832

In a time of rapid development of the professions and concomitant specialization, of challenges to existing religious beliefs and renegotiation of political and class oppositions, the arrival of the cholera meant the commencement of a struggle over the location and sources of the authority to define its meanings.[1] Indeed, in this period, every political question (as cholera rapidly came to be defined) was debated also as a religious question; as historian Eileen Groth Lyon points out, conservatives, radicals, and everyone in between had their own take on the relevance of the scripture to current conflicts (77). However, such questions now invited the input of a new kind of more secular expert as well. This struggle overlapped with, and sometimes was contained within, other struggles of longer standing, but epidemics, like other dramatic public events, have a way of forcing such disputes to crisis. In official and unofficial bulletins, pamphlets, reports, sermons, and articles, Anglican clergy and the emerging medical profession struggled over the right to publicly interpret the social meanings of cholera.[2] This conflict over social authority exposes the ways in which discourses of national identity were being mobilized throughout the mid-nineteenth century. By the end of the period, a partial redrawing of the boundaries between the two "camps," but also a partial erosion of those boundaries occurs; the "disaggregation of domains" of knowledge and authority, as theorist Mary Poovey elaborates, is neither a simple nor linear process.

In the early days of the first (1832) epidemic, cholera was believed to be the special scourge of the impious and dissolute. Cholera would strike those who scorned the Sabbath, who drank and blasphemed, and who mocked the illness as the expression of God's anger (the literature abounds with examples of people who laugh at the cholera—often, not coincidentally, in pubs—and are stricken "that very night!"). The poor were hardest hit, thus confirming the general perception that poverty was the result of sin, and a kind of sin itself. Clergy and medics both shaped public perception of the epidemic: the clergy as the official and state-sanctioned arbiter of morality and the medics as part of an emerging area of public administration officially represented by hastily thrown together "boards of health," delegated by the Privy Council mid-epidemic, with uncertain powers and even more limited credibility.

Additionally, the boards and those clergy who tried to assist them faced a recalcitrant public in the midst of reform agitation, sceptical of the existence of cholera as a disease and inclined to lump together clergy and medical authorities with Tory and capitalist interests. No one has undertaken to look very specifically at the clerical reaction to the epidemic, especially in published sermons. However, an impressive number of sermons were published in response to the epidemic, which had a wide audience and a powerful, even definitive impact on how the issues of cholera and public health were framed. Close examination suggests that there were specific historical and political reasons that conservative, pro-establishment Anglican churchmen, who authored the majority of these sermons, reacted to cholera in the way they did—that is, to declare cholera in Britain a national emergency brought on by national sin (when it was, after all, a world pandemic).[3] This framing of the cholera reflected specific challenges to the authority of the church in this period, including political but also religious reform, and the emerging power of a newly institutionalized scientific discourse. In short, the articulation of the cholera epidemic as public discourse had as much or more to do with the vicissitudes of a particular historical moment as with the prevailing intellectual understanding of disease.

Careful examination of these materials, not only in their individual political contexts, but in dialogue with each other, shows how cholera became a foundational political issue itself. It contributed to the targeting of public health in what came to be called the "Condition of England" question, in the struggle of the lower classes for inclusion in the national body, indeed, in the very definition and identification of nation with a middle-class, clean, British body, which, by the 1850s, would become racialized as specifically white and English. It did so, in part, because vocal pro-establishment churchmen (that is, those opposed to any separation between the church and the state, who saw the church as the guide of the state rather than its subordinate) used cholera as a platform for their identification of the church as the nation's teacher in such a way as to set the terms for the debate throughout different interest groups. For the remainder of the period, charitable, housing, and labor reform would focus on health, above all other issues, as that which bound the "two nations" into a single body through a communicative medium of disease. The confluence of discourses emerging from the church crisis and reform with the chronological accident of the cholera epidemic led to specific discursive moves on the part of church, state, medical authorities, and labor organizations. In turn, these moves caused images and metaphors particular to the circumstances of the first cholera epidemic to gain an important, even constitutive, force in the discourse of the national body as it emerged over the next four decades.

Before the cholera epidemic became a public issue, the crisis of reform had already inspired calls for a collective fast emphasizing diminishing national unity. The "crisis" had not only to do with the first Reform Bill per se, but with the momentous events of the late 1820s that had preceded it and were representative of the same spirit, especially the elimination of Catholic disabilities and the repeal of the Test and Corporations Acts.[4] These legislative actions enabled some non-Anglican Christians (especially Catholics) to have more direct political representation and indeed, to hold public office. Since, as Linda Colley notes, the idea of Britain as a "nation" depended more on Protestantism than on, say, ethnicity, it is unsurprising that these changes were seen by many as an erosion of the integrity of national unity. Within the Church of England, establishmentarians indignantly prophesied doom.[5] Perhaps the most famous response was "National Apostasy," John Keble's 1833 Assize Sermon:

> Omens and tokens of an Apostate Mind in a nation . . . [include a most alarming symptom:] the growing indifference, in which men indulge themselves, to other men's religious sentiments. Under the guise of charity and toleration we are come almost to this pass; that no difference, in matters of faith, is to disqualify for our approbation. . . . I do not speak of public measures only. . . . But I speak of the spirit which leads men to exult in every step of that kind; to congratulate one another on the supposed decay of what they call an exclusive system. . . . Is it not saying . . . "we will be as the heathen," the aliens to the Church of our Redeemer? (127–33)

This ill-intentioned "spirit which leads men" was the spirit of reform, which extended beyond the recognition of Irish Catholics to the recognition of £10 householders enfranchised in 1832.[6] Many of these were very likely to be dissenters, especially in the industrial North, the Midlands, and the West, where the Anglican Church was not as strong as in the agricultural South.[7] Much of Keble's sermon focuses on the church's loss of its privileged status and its legislative power, and this is specifically couched in a rhetoric of alienation—to become "as the heathens, the aliens" within one's own nation.

Keble's reference to charity is particularly charged. The charity and tolerance that had been urged in favor of Catholic emancipation was textually based on Corinthians 12, wherein the church is defined as a single body made of many members with differing talents and views. Charity is urged as the antidote to doctrinal and personal squabbling that will violate the body's unity. But for Keble, the body invoked was not that of Christianity broadly conceived, but of the Anglican Church per se. Many calls to unity, both those addressed to clergy and those addressed to congregations, emphasized this body metaphor, and identified it with the body of the nation—a body that itself was being rearticulated through reform. This body was clearly not only the Christian community, it was also the state that represented it. For Keble, supporting an established church, the church was coterminous with both nation and state. Keble worried that extending the body to encompass "alien" beliefs would shatter its unity.

The politically conservative secular community as well framed reform as a disaster of national proportions and as a degeneration of the social body. As early as February 15, 1831, well before the advent of cholera, the *Times* reported MP Spencer Perceval's parliamentary motion for a general fast: "The state of the country loudly called for a measure like his—that it was in a state of political and religious disorganization—that the elements of its constitution were hourly being loosened;— . . . corruption was showing its face, and the body corporate was diseased from head to foot." In fact, the motion was at this time withdrawn. However, when the cholera finally did arrive a year later, "a national day of fasting and humiliation" was finally declared in Parliament, legitimating the religious action as an affair of state.

Naturally, such an occasion invited reflection on the individual's relationship to the nation, particularly in terms of the rhetoric of the epidemic and its focus on the individual culpability of cholera victims. The official liturgy of the Church of England insisted on national guilt and sinfulness; in Hull, local clergy excerpted the prayer and printed it in a penny tract, along with a text that catechized the reader, who was assumed to be reluctant to admit to sin and had to be prodded to do so. Such fast days were declared in times of any national calamity, including war and famine; however, on no similar occasion in the period have I found an outpouring of literature as voluble and dramatic on the subject of national sin as this one.[8] Believing the church was facing spoilation, and according to some alarmists, disestablishment, many felt the church was in its most serious political crisis since the interregnum. Church of England conservatives were highly motivated to identify the church forcefully with the nation, and to emphasize its role as instructor to the people and interpreter of their collective experiences.[9]

The Church of England liturgy insisted on the guilt of the nation. Yet the public was also often told that the disease would only strike those *individuals* who were sinful and intemperate. By the end of the epidemic, there was some attempt to decriminalize the victims, or at least admit that not all cholera victims were drunkards and, in any case, must be treated as patients rather than reprobates. Still, the language wavered between a careful neutrality and blame. For example, Charles Gaselee and Alexander Tweedie, authors of *A Practical Treatise on the Cholera*, admit that after the first wave of epidemic, when "It fell principally, almost wholly, on the lower classes of society. . . . In June it returned; all parts of London, and most of the Suburbs, felt its influence: the city was severely visited; all ranks of life became affected . . . the assurances of the security of the affluent, have proved to be erroneous and futile" (2). However, the anonymous author of "Why Are You Afraid of the Cholera?" gives calm, technical medical directions, in the midst of which, apropos of nothing obvious, the author bursts out: "The greater part of those who have died of the cholera have been bad, dirty, drunken and idle people!" (By the Author . . . 8). The *Working Man's Companion*, published by the SDUK, temporized, "On the one hand, a large majority of persons who have died of cholera have been very poor and wretched, and disposed to disease by the weakness that poor living has occasioned. This is no time to remind any of them, poor people, that their poverty has come of their idleness, or that their poor diet might be better if they were not extravagant and not ignorant" (161). It goes on to warn its intended audience of mechanics and artisans, which is quite carefully separated from the population thus described, that *any* kind of intemperance could bring on the cholera—not just alcohol, but excessive eating, not eating enough, or eating too much of one kind of food. On the whole, the attitude of the English basically coincided with that of the French medic Amedee

Lefevre, whom George Rees, M.D., cites as an authority on the disease: "'There is this peculiarity in the Cholera, it attacks the dissolute and the drunkard . . . it was observed to clear the towns it invaded [in Persia] of all such as . . . were a nuisance to society.'" To which Rees adds, "Who can tell then what advantages may ultimately arise from that which we now so painfully anticipate? That which is now the object of our fears, may hereafter be the subject of our gratitude" (Rees 34–35).

It is hardly odd, then, that the clergy faced difficulties making their congregations feel responsible for and unified with the victims of the first epidemic. Clergyman James A. Taylor runs through a veritable catalog of sins, apparently hoping that every auditor would have felt guilty of *something*.

> How does the nation at large profane the *Day* of the Lord, instead of *remembering* to "keep it holy!" How generally is it made a day of business, of feasting, of pleasure, of excess, of a double tide of sin! How is it desecrated by the issue of Newspapers, which, in righteous judgement for the national sin of permitting such a violation of God's law, circulate principles of insubordination, immorality and vice! Are not shops opened and encouraged for the sale of avowed infidel publications: while the sabbath has its licensed lecturers in infidelity! How does whoredom pollute the land! How disgraceful to common decency is the state of our streets! How is the papacy . . . nationally cherished! While 800,000 of our fellow beings are still held in slavery! (12–13)

Taylor continues to list other possibilities: dissipation of the great, discontent of the lower orders with their own position, and drunkenness are added to the list of national sins. He then covers anything he might have forgotten, "These are things, with many others which might be named, which form a mass of increasing national guilt" (13). He concludes, "Lastly, forget not our guilty country. Individually, in your families, in your public assembly, most humbly confess before Almighty God the nation's guilt and its worthiness to suffer" (Taylor 33).

In this fairly typical sermon, there is a clear concern with mediating between the units of subnational groups—the individual, the family, the public assembly—and the larger entity of nation. There is also the usual concern with non-Anglican religion (the "licensed lecturers in infidelity" are probably Catholics, as attack on the papacy is a strong theme in this sermon, though they might also simply be dissenters). Taylor suggests that sins in "public" spaces—"whoredom," "the state of our streets," "licensed lecturers," and "Newspapers"—are more chargeable as national sins than crimes regularly committed in "private" spaces. Who is committing these sins is also not entirely clear: "permitting" the sale of newspapers is presumably the responsibility of government, but "drunkenness" is the sin of an individual, though augmented by its presence in public space.

Probably most clergy were less concerned with the theoretical issues of the individual's relationship to the nation than they were with impressing upon their flocks that such a connection surely existed. The local clergy of Newcastle-upon-Tyne put together a small pamphlet of which they distributed twenty thousand free copies. In it, they explain that all disease is sent by God in punishment of sin, and that many sins are committed by many daily, "But the question again returns, WHAT SIN SO PREVAILS IN THIS TOWN AND NEIGHBORHOOD AS TO BE CONSIDERED THE CAUSE OF THIS PESTILENCE?" ("An Affectionate Address" 3). The authors offer no clear answer to this question, instead offering anecdotes of sinners stricken by cholera. In this catalog, however, there is again a suggestion that public spectacle involves sin that "spreads" to spectators, much as the countenancing (and perhaps even reading) of newspapers in Taylor's text causes public culpability:

> About noon on Christmas Day, (which was also the Holy Sabbath!) in the lower part of the Town and in Bottle Bank, such scenes of drunkenness and outrage were witnessed, as would be disgraceful in a heathen country. Men and women were staggering in a state of complete intoxication. Some were brawling and fighting, while crowds were collected as spectators to glory in their shame. The streets in this case were almost impassable. (5)

Cholera, Taylor emphasizes, struck the community that same night (5). National identity (set against the "heathen" country) is betrayed by the spectators who "glory" in the shame of their fellow subjects—though it might seem impossible to avoid stopping to witness such a spectacle, the streets being "impassable." In this and many other tracts or sermons relating to the national fast day, clergy returned again and again to the issue of national versus individual sin, suggesting a need to make sense of a relationship that was rather unclear to their audience, if not themselves.

Anglican clergy were thus placed in a peculiar position. While confirming that cholera was punishment for individual sin, and agreeing with medical reassurances to the public that those who lived more wholesomely would be spared, they were also in the difficult position of dealing with the stricken individual as part of a larger body, a national population. Thus, clergy were faced with the task of negotiating between a concept of individual sinfulness and the cholera as a specifically national punishment. The middle classes to whom such sermons were largely addressed were exhorted over the course of the century to feel socially responsible for the plight of the poor and to envision themselves and the poor as parts of a unified and responsible nation. But these social classes also tended to categorize themselves as separate from the very poor and sick, who were alternately seen as a festering illness in the social body and a foreign threat intruding upon it.

OTHER CLERICAL RESPONSES, 1832–1867

The burden of the Anglican clergy in England was, in this way, unique.[10] Although many religious groups seemed to have joined in observance of the national fast day—on the day of Humiliation, medic and historian Thomas Shapter records that the Jewish synagogue, the Roman Catholic Church, the dissenting chapels, and the Anglican churches "were alike open, and crowded by attentive congregations" (254)—they did not all respond discursively in the same ways. Catholics in England laid low, published little on the causes of the cholera, and contented themselves with ministering to their flock, who were largely represented among the classes most affected.[11] Mass Irish emigration in the late 1840s from famine-struck Ireland also brought the usual responses to penurious immigrants, and was not improved by the typhus epidemic that attended the overcrowded Irish poor. The fact that these newcomers were largely Catholic did nothing to improve English attitudes toward Catholicism. Even as late as 1866, philanthropist Catherine Marsh, in a highly fictionalized account of cholera wards in which dying people burst spontaneously into hymns, concludes her tract with the "proven fact" that Rome is identical with Babylon:

> Earnest Christians! to whom the truth of God is precious, and scarcely less precious your freedom to teach it to others—Protestant Christians! . . . Englishmen! who by the nobleness of nature God has given you, love the daylight of true English Institutions, without veil, vow, or mystery—awake to the danger of your religion and your country—with the resolve of "NO SURRENDER TO ROME!" If ever the saying were true, it is true for each one of you now, "NEUTRALITY IS TREASON,"—treason against the honour of your God—treason against the liberties of your land. (68–69)

In fact, often the sin most strongly hinted to be the deciding factor in God's wrath was England's tolerance of Catholicism—this could spill over even to ritualist forms of Anglicanism. G. Huelin notes that Anglican Bishop Jacobson was pelted with mud by "Orangemen" in Liverpool after blessing a cholera hospital because he put sisters in charge of it. The crowd yelled "Down with the old Puseyite Bishop!" (Huelin 138).[12]

The Methodists, by contrast, provide a good example of how a major dissenting group handled the epidemic. Although I have no comparable Methodist sermons to refer to (perhaps because they were not preserved or published, and were more often delivered extemporaneously than their Anglican counterparts), the treatment of the cholera epidemics in the *Wesleyan Methodist Magazine*, published in London, is quite different than that in Anglican sermons. Its first significant response came in 1832. Although the magazine took up the cry of a national sin in the first epidemic, it completely dropped the topic after that. Further, even in the first epidemic, writers for the *Wesleyan* utilized the rhetoric of the Anglicans against the established church:

> The present state of Great Britain is calculated to awaken deep anxiety in the breast of every Christian patriot. The Legislature is divided upon a question of great interest. . . . The sufferings of the poor are severe and extensive. A spirit of lawless riot is gone forth. . . . A pestilence, which has spread deso-lation over extensive islands and continents, which baffles the efforts of sci-ence and humanity . . . has already made its appearance in the Northern part of the island . . . no power but God can arrest its progress and cause it to dis-appear. . . . Should the pestilence become general, in addition to distress occasioned by the breaking of families, there will be an increased stagnation of trade, and consequent aggravation of the sufferings of the poor; and the resources of our public charities will be in a great measure dried up. The increase of crime is appalling; the national wickedness is great;—its guilt is enhanced . . . by the religious privileges which have been so long enjoyed and so grievously abused. . . . [The people] have to take the lead in humiliation and prayer; and to use, on behalf of a guilty land, that "power with God." ("Didymus," "Weekly Intercession Meeting" 12–15)

Here one sees the appeal to a "patriotic Christian" national identity of the "people" and the association of the disease with the "lawless" rioting of polit-ical protest. However, the national sin is *not* that of "the people" but of the established religious leadership. It is the people who must intercede with God on behalf of the guilty land. And of course, part of the sin is precisely the enjoyment of establishment prerogatives. Further, the poor are simply to be compassionated, not blamed, and the responsibility even for poverty may lie elsewhere.

"Didymus" was the only author in the *Wesleyan* who consistently tack-led the "national sin" issue. On the occasion of the public fast, he says that God is indeed responsible for the "chastisement," noting that "Nations, as such, have no existence in eternity [unlike individuals]. . . . Wicked nations, therefore are always punished in the present world" ("The Public Fast" 258).[13] (Innocent individuals, he assures his readers, will be compensated by God in the next life.) He emphasizes the efficacy of individual prayer (as opposed to the Anglican emphasis on group/national prayer) on behalf of *others*. Again, the parishioner is not the responsible party. The sins named are slavery in the West Indies, Sabbath profanation, infidelity to Christian-ity (here defined broadly as Christian values), the suffering of the poor, and finally, and most importantly, judging by the space given to it, *lack* of reli-gious toleration.

> While Christians of different denominations are conflicting with each other
> on account of their minor differences, and criminally endeavoring to weaken
> each other's influence, the enemy is actively employed in sowing the tares of
> infidelity and revolution; population has increased beyond all former exam-
> ple; and for a vast proportion of the people no religious instruction has been
> provided. These proceedings cannot but be displeasing to the Almighty
> God. (262)

This passage both recognizes that the Anglican church is using the epidemic
for political purposes and condemns it—though the author goes on to use the
cholera for his own political purposes in turn. It takes up the rhetoric seen
later in sanitary texts (the Malthusian rhetoric of overpopulation, for example). But it also turns the establishmentarians' claim that religious diversity is
fostering revolution on its head, suggesting that it is the refusal to countenance religious diversity that spawns "infidelity" (here to faith, rather than a
particular church) and revolution.

In February 1832, also in the *Wesleyan*, an anonymous author writes,
"God has a controversy with us. The national burdens are evidently too great
for the . . . British empire. The country faints under its enormous load of debt
and national expenditure" ("Retrospective of Public Affairs" 151). He warns
that if political struggle should "arise, and noxious humours of the body politic
grow" to spawn revolution, that there is a newly impoverished population,
who, although well educated and accustomed to comfort, are now disaffected
and nearly indigent. This group, he states, "would be both disposed and qual-
ified to effect . . . mischief; and even under more favourable circumstances, the
rapid increase of such a class of society, with the continually extending pau-
perization of multitudes of labourers and artisans, cannot be sufficiently
deplored" ("Retrospective of Public Affairs" 151). Here the national sin is bad
financial management, and a punitive system of poor relief, rather than the
individual sins of the people. In short, these are economic and political evils,
not violations of the commandments and certainly not apostasy.

The national and political bodies are not necessarily the same in this text,
although there is clearly some relation between them: the nation is "burdened"
economically, which creates the result of the body politic's potential illness.
The body politic could contain within itself an enemy of the nation: a newly
pauperized but intelligent out-group that might or might not be part of the
nation per se. It was precisely the economic domain that slipped between the
social and the political; in a free market, economics were supposed to operate
autonomous of politics, as a self-regulating system much like the healthy body
itself. Poovey claims that between the 1830s and '40s, the "social sphere . . .
had come to mirror the economic domain" (11). Certainly, the economic was
felt to be a measure of the health of the nation, not identical with the social

body, but closely aligned with it. Timothy Alborn has charted the use of epidemiological metaphors to define economic crises in this period, such as defining bank panics as "the Asiatic cholera of the commercial world" (282).[14] As Alborn points out, "intemperate" speculators were faced with the same Malthusian retributive God, who "unfailingly delivered pestilence as a positive check to working-class population growth" (283).

In the *Wesleyan*, the cholera was credited as a means of grace in some cases of deathbed conversions (Sugden 819–20). Further, unlike the relatively rare mentions of cholera deaths within the Anglican community (often the cause of death was hidden), the *Wesleyan* was full of obituaries in 1832 that record cholera as the cause of death of pious, respectable people. Later issues do not mention the cholera as a religious issue at all, nor do they connect disease to national identity. Further, unlike the Anglicans, the Methodists mention France's epidemic with sympathy and suggest prayer for them. Like the Catholics' claims in France, Anglicans' claims that cholera was punishment for a specifically national sin of infidelity were weakened by the fact that cholera was a world pandemic, a fact that the government of France did not fail to point out to the Catholic Bishops (Delaporte).

R. J. Morris is the only scholar to date who has devoted considerable space to the discussion of the religious response in Britain in 1832. He identifies the common ground of the diverse clergy who responded to the cholera-sin equation as evangelicism; he sees them as making a fairly homogenous connection across the board between sin and divine vengeance in the cholera. Because he does not examine the role of reform or of nation, he misses some of the differences between pro-establishment Anglican evangelicals and dissenting evangelicals. He focuses only on the theological underpinnings of this attitude, and the one difference he does cite—that the lower down the social status scale the leadership of a religious group was, the more specific the sin was for which one was punished (154)—is explained in reference to the specific needs and habits of parishioners. For example, he notes that drink was a severe sin for Methodists because among the working classes drink might make the difference between comfortable survival and penury. This is a useful observation, but it seems clear upon further examination that the political issues of establishment and attitude toward reform also had a great deal to do with the way sins were described, especially whether cholera was defined as retribution for national sins or personal ones, although Morris does mention that the Methodists used the cholera to attack the established church's attitude toward dissent (133).

Additionally, because Morris's study is limited to 1832, he does not follow the further development of this discourse in subsequent epidemics, and so does not pay attention to the way the topic falls out of Methodist discourse after the 1832 epidemic. Morris very usefully observes, however, the tendency of rural dissenting groups to hold revivals during cholera epidemics that depended heavily upon a rhetoric of self accusation (144–46). Although these seem to have been more directed toward personal than national guilt, it is difficult to gauge the extent to which they might have used the language of the establishment, since they published no tracts documenting their generally unscripted sermons. As Morris states, the "traditional Anglican" was often disturbed by the "dangerous enthusiasm" of the evangelicals, who would "make religion a matter of personal contact between man and his God, without the necessary intervention of the State and the traditional structures of the Church" (145). It is this representation that works against the overarching corporative response that the "national sin" rhetoric fostered. Charles Kingsley, Anglican minister and enlightened sanitarian, attacked the cholera-is-punishment attitude as barbarous and dangerous, heightening fear and exposure to illness rather than conserving the health and energy of the people. He associates this rhetoric with dissenting evangelical fringe groups. But the same charge was made against the established church by many medics in the mid-century epidemics of 1849–1855, and, as previously shown, the rhetoric of many Anglican sermons indeed blames the sinner, although simultaneously making gestures toward a corporate guilt. It is hard to say clearly what sect, if any, with which this attitude would have been most particularly associated.

Morris found evidence of only one Methodist cholera revival in 1854 (in Cornwall), at which "God the Avenger" still played a significant role (203). However, such rhetoric is common enough long before the cholera epidemics, and afterward, that one need not assume itinerant preachers were borrowing from Anglican evangelicals. It is highly probable, however, that these preachers were not making the same connections between establishment and the nation upon which the Anglican rhetoric depended so heavily. In short, like political radicals, Methodists used the existing rhetorical framework given by the hegemonic power for defining the epidemic. They then used it to contest that power by redefining meanings within the original explanatory structure for their own ends (e.g., the sin was sectarian intolerance, rather than infidelity or reform). They were also quicker to abandon this framework when it was not useful, and to use it to indict the powerful rather than to build national identity among their own parishioners. Establishmentarian Anglicans tried to include their congregations under a sense of national sinfulness, whereas the Methodists were more likely to warn their flock against individual sins, and cite national sins as those of Anglican clergy and Tory MPs. Thus, the initial religious response to the cholera in 1832 varied, but the responses coalesced around questions of sin and responsibility, national and minority identities. The second epidemic, however, would see considerably more complication in the responses, and a new group claiming a right to speak publicly about cholera and its meanings: medics.

2

After 1832

Medical Authority and the Clergy

BY THE SECOND EPIDEMIC IN 1848, many Anglican clergy were embattled, not only with the popular perception of cholera as a "filth disease," which was a class rather than a national issue, but also with the rapidly growing medical profession. Medics' tendency to see disease as largely a physical affair divested it of its moral significance—or, at least, shifted morality to the care of the body and the relationship with the self and the environment, rather than the relationship with God. Stripped of its original political context, the rhetoric a new generation of clergy inherited from the first epidemic seventeen years before positioned them against the medical profession, which had gained considerably in power and credibility during that time.

The sense of the specificity of sins for which the nation was accountable—and for which parishioners were likely to feel a collective responsibility—was even less defined in the second epidemic than the first. On the Sunday appointed for the national fast in 1849, English evangelical and anti-Tractarian Edward Bickersteth (1786–1850), then rector of Watton, wrote, "Sin, our national and our personal sin, is the cause of this. . . . There is very considerable danger of our losing sight of this, by looking only at second things in which its special power is manifested: such as accumulated filth, want of drainage, unhealthy diet, and the like. . . . But these things have existed in other years" (2). Spiritual, physical, and economic health are conflated in a single "national" body:[1] "Heavy judgements have fallen upon our country. The year 1847, and subsequent years have been disastrous in our mercantile annals. Losses by depreciation of funded property, and in railway shares, and in West India produce, and in Colonial property, it has been calculated, have amounted to several hundred millions" (Bickersteth 4). Punishments, it appears, could be economic, as well as epidemic.

Bickersteth also offers a laundry list of sins:

> The same fearful sins of INTENSE WORLDLINESS, EXTENDED SABBATH-BREAKING, LUXURY, OPPRESSION OF THE POOR, LAWLESS INSUBORDINATION, INFIDELITY, NEGLECTED SPIRITUAL INTERESTS OF OUR FELLOW MEN, NEGLECT OF GOD AND HIS TRUTH IN OUR PUBLIC JOURNALS AND POPULAR LITERATURE still prevail and extend among us. We have still to say, OUR VAST COLONIAL EMPIRE, a most responsible trust . . . HAS NOT BEEN DULY USED FOR GOD AND HIS GLORY; but has been chiefly used for gaining wealth and aggrandizing our country . . . THE SINS OF THE CHURCH OF CHRIST, in the apostasy of some of its ministers to Rome . . . have also to be confessed. (4)

Finally, after these "widespread" sins (often sins of omission), he concludes, "We have each also personal sins. . . . All our transgressions of God's law, and all our abuse or neglect of his gospel, make a part of the national guilt, and add to its amount" (5). Bickersteth has certainly covered all the bases. One still senses an unease regarding the exact nature of the specifically national sin that caused cholera, although once again the press comes in for a share of the blame, indicating a widespread perception that the public sphere of print culture was the *fons et*, perhaps, *origo* of an important component of national shared culture and therefore identity.[2] Philip Bland's sermon at St. Mary's, Rotherhithe, simply refuses to name sins; clearly there had been a sin and the proof is in the pestilence; therefore, he concludes, parishioners should simply meditate on their own sins with a wholesome fear of God's wrath (8). William Braithwaite, in preaching to a rural congregation at Bideford, cautions against identifying particular sins with individuals, leading to uncharity.

> It is, then, neither of right nor of love, to look upon all misfortunes which befall men, as judgements or punishments for sin. In the case of individual sufferers, it can seldom be safe to do so. Who are we, that we should judge others? And yet it is also most true, that, as in the case of nations and multitudes, so too of individuals, God's manifest judgement has often overtaken the sin, and overwhelmed the evil-doer. . . . There is, however, less fear in mistaking, and certainly less danger to ourselves in considering national chastisements as judgements for national sins. (5–6)

This offers a much more charitable attitude toward individual sin and suffering than in the first epidemic. Braithwaite is mindful of the potential misuses of such a doctrine, leading to unchristian judgment of others. Unfortunately, he points out, God is undiscriminating regarding individual sinners once guilt "goes national": "in national judgements, it is not only the guilty who suffer, or only the innocent who escape" (11). He suggests that the cities are the source of national sin, but "God is angry with our land. . . . The pestilence is in the land" (11). In Bideford, "There may not, indeed, be the gross hideousness of sin which stalks abroad in our largest towns. . . . God forbid that such should come among us! Alas for our nation, when such shall begin to show themselves beyond their breeding places, and wander out into the green fields and quiet dwelling places of our land!" (11). Innocent rural populations suffer for the guilt of "our largest towns," and the exact sin goes unnamed, as the nation becomes a population conflated with a certain geography. This sermon is unusual, however, since it asks for contrition from its audience, yet indicates that the real sinners are elsewhere, in the city. The Reverend D. F. Jarman, in a threepenny tract, also insists on an unspecified sin as the root cause of disease: "It is no fable . . . sin is the very root and cause of cholera. We never would have found it in this land had there not been some flagrant guilt to punish. . . . Whatever may be the *apparent* cause, this is the *real* cause" (6). What this flagrant guilt may be cannot be named (though he hints it may be apostasy within the church) because, in fact, he doesn't know what it is: "now there is some alarming increase to our national guilt . . . it is our duty, with the Spirit's aid, to search it out. Oh for skill to find it!" (8).

THE MEDICAL RESPONSE

Meanwhile, medics for the first time publicly attacked the church's right to define the social causes of cholera, staking out the body and public health as their own turf. Forbes Winslow, physician and influential psychological specialist, argued both in the *Morning Chronicle* and in a tract reprint of the same letter that "Fear is the predisposing cause of plague" (5), and suggested that calming the public and preserving general good spirits was far more important than denouncing sins. And an exasperated individual identified only as Sensus Communis attacked the language of the Church of England liturgy directly, arguing that, although, the prayer that congregations had been ordered to speak, "on the assumption that this grievous disease comes directly from the hand of the Almighty as a *special judgement* on the nation for its guilt" had been legitimized by very weighty authorities, it was simply wrong. The writer summarizes, "In the public employment of this prayer, millions of devout men have been led to imply their positive belief in two very remarkable propositions"— first, that cholera is sent by God as punishment, and second, that 'humiliation and repentance' shall avert it (3–4). Regarding the prevailing set of opinions with respect to poverty and the church's position on it, Sensus Communis writes, "I know that Britain's wealth is often adduced as an evidence of Britain's worth in the sight of God . . . [but] I deny that with nations, any more than with individuals, there is any necessary connexion between their worldly prosperity and their spiritual purity" (7–8). He further points out that the church's position is implicitly hostile to sanitary reform: "Does it not in effect tell them [the poor] that what the doctors tell them . . . about the danger of want of cleanliness, and the deadly effects of vice and intemperance, is sheer nonsense? . . . that *it is the hand of GOD, and not their filthy condition*" (12–13).

In this powerful tract, the author challenges the church on three key premises: first, that neither "national calamities" nor "national blessings" are to be interpreted morally—in short, by the church; second, that the tie between individual prosperity and health and national prosperity and health—precisely the connection the church tries to strengthen in its assertion of national guilt—is untenable; and finally, that the authority of the clergy is misused when it challenges the more rightful authority of medicine. His choice of pseudonym is telling. Playing on the pun of "common sense," he actually arrogates to himself the vox populi as the "collective knowledge or feeling of the community." He implies that the church's ability to speak for Britain was limited, not only by lack of common sense, but by lack of fellowship or common cause with the people (although he or she also speaks of the poor in the third person). Sensus Communis also points out the logical inconsistency of commonly held—and church reinforced—beliefs about class, culpability, and disease with the church's attempt to unify its parishioners in experiencing responsibility for the epidemic.

Although there was little direct public commentary by the medical profession on the church's position during the first epidemic, there were already hostilities between some medics and the Tory establishment that included the Anglican Church, then very vulnerable to critique from a number of sources. *The Lancet*, for example, at the forefront of the battle for professional standing for medics, was quite proreform under the editorship of radical Thomas Wakley (1795–1862), and equated medical reform (improvement and clarification of professional knowledge, standards and training) with political reform, which it designated specifically as "National Improvement" (2). A four-page polemic by the editors in 1831–1832 attacked the church openly on the occasion of the traditional toast to the king at a medical society dinner being amended to the older "To the Church and King": "The Church-and-King conclave lost no opportunities of raising obstacles to the progress of knowledge generally. . . . The Church and King *system* [original emphasis], whatever may have been its advantages to the clergy, has proved a terrible bane to the mass of the people of England, and a bitter curse to the members of the medical profession" (Wakley, 220–21).

Clearly, it would be an error to read this as exemplary of all medics. Wakley, a surgeon and (from 1835–1852) Member of Parliament for Finsbury, was a well-known radical. Still the *Lancet* was a powerful (if abrasive) voice for professionalization (and leveling and unification of the profession). For the middle-class readers of the *Lancet*, the antireform Tories not only represented aristocratic elitism, but also a hatred of the scientific and positivist values that were fundamental to both science and the concept of professionalism. This belief is evident in the rhetoric of the other medical attacks on the clerical position as well. Many of these were written by a few medics who were politically radical, and may not have represented a majority opinion, (as might also be said of the Anglicans who wrote most prolifically on the cholera). Still, they were vocal minorities, and it is through their agency and from their perspective the issues were introduced to the public eye. From the perspective of the public, then, these may have seemed to be more broadly representative of a schism between the two authorities than, perhaps, they were.

The *Lancet* was an outspoken and jealous defender of the professional prerogatives and authority of medical men. It was the first to attack, however fairly, the first Board of Health for not including more medical professionals. It also took the board to task for the regulations and recommendations the board issued regarding cholera treatment. On August 25, 1832, although it applauded the recommendations of the board generally, the *Lancet* chided the board for giving the public instructions for treating the disease. Instead, noted the editors, patients should be advised to have immediate recourse to medical advice and not to self-medicate: "medical skills should be resorted to as the *only* rock to which the unhappy patient can cling with any hope of temporary redemption or permanent security" (The *Lancet* 1831–1832, 2:657). In an era of official anti-contagionism, it also took the anti-trade position that cholera was spread by human activity.[3]

Meanwhile, other religious and philanthropic religious organizations, although basically in agreement with the church about the status of cholera as a divine message, began also in their access to print to pose a threat to Church of England supremacy simply by printing opinions that could be read as contradicting doctrine. The *London City Mission Magazine*, in October 1849, reinstitutes the boundaries between lower-class sinners and the middle classes, even while countering the claims of medics to place the guilt of cholera on sanitary conditions rather than individual actions:

> Looking, as we ought to do, beyond second causes in such a matter as this, and regarding the disease as sent from God, in the way of chastisement for our offenses . . . it naturally leads to the inquiry, whether or not the *peculiar* neglect of God, so common among the working classes, may not have been connected with the especials ingling [*sic*] out of these classes for the

judgement. . . . For there can be no question that they, *as a class*, in our metropolis, have given far less heed to the soul than other orders of individuals. ("The Cholera and Its Effects . . ." 205)

Founded in 1835 by David Nasmith, the mission was a nondenominational, evangelical project dedicated to the urban poor in a moment when the Anglican church was criticized for caring only for the wealthy. In this text, cholera is a judgment on a population, rather than individuals. But the population is identified by class, rather than as a nation, which works against the rhetoric of the state church. Subsequently, the article attacks "authorities" (i.e., the Board of Health) for attending to the needs of the body, while the needs of the soul are not being looked to, but indicts the church also for its well-known disregard of the lower classes. The church and the Boards of Health, then, were the official and visible leaders of two large camps, each riven within itself with conflicts, but each forming a group with common cause against the "misguided officiousness" of the other group. This conflict—between two duly appointed authorities, each representing, in its own way, the crown—was to come to a crisis in the third epidemic, just four years later, in which Lord Palmerston (Henry John Temple) declined to propose the usual fast in Parliament, in favor of more energetic sanitary measures.[4]

The third cholera epidemic had not yet arrived in England when Lord Palmerston's secretary penned his courteous but firm rejection of the fast-day proposal, suggesting that a national fast was less appropriate than using the time before spring to make civic improvements in impoverished neighborhoods, "which, if allowed to remain [unaltered], will infallibly breed pestilence, and be fruitful in death, in spite of all the prayers and fastings of an united but inactive nation. When man has done his utmost for his own safety then it is time to invoke the blessing of Heaven." The response to Palmerston was immediate and indignant, although interestingly the most inflammatory response came from outside the Anglican church, which was by then beginning to position itself closer to the sanitarians. The Scottish Presbyterian Reverend Robert Buchanan's response is exemplary of the most extreme rhetoric. He charges Palmerston with irresponsibility: "In an age especially like this—an age prone to physical rather than metaphysical science—an age essentially materialistic in its spirit and pursuits . . . the whole problem of such a visitation as the cholera is solved without respect to any moral cause or object whatsoever—whether in the character and conduct of men, or in the purposes of God. Mere material agencies and influences explain it all" (14–17). Describing Palmerston's position as one of "gross materialism," he complains that "Material pollutions are held as the sole provocatives of the cholera. . . . It can need little argument to show that this is a representation as shallow as it is pernicious" (14–17). However, in order to argue against this materialism, Buchanan finds it necessary to attack the sanitary project as well, arguing that people *choose* to be filthy *because* they are evil, and radically distancing the "nation" from the criminalized poor, and by extension, from potential cholera victims:

> Our statesmen and civil governors are almost at their wits' end to know what to do with that refuse and scum of society which is continually boiling up from the depths in which it is gendered, and running over upon the rest of the community. Our colonies will no longer have this foul residuum drained off from Great Britain, and poured out upon them. Deprived of this outlet, our bursting prisons and penitentiaries are now, it seems, to be periodically opened, and ticket-of-leave convicts . . . are to be let loose. (36)

Buchanan displaces the "sanitary" evil from the sewers onto the "moral" evil of the populace, which itself becomes a moral and physical sanitation problem. This "residuum" of the population is outside the nation and beyond reclamation—the question is simply what to do with it without an "outlet."

This rhetoric is entangled with the sanitary discourse surrounding overfilled cemeteries, which were receiving particular attention in this period. In fact, public attention had shifted, in part because of successful sanitary efforts since 1848, from the visible sanitary problem of the refuse of the living (e.g., dunghills above ground) to the invisible problems to be found immediately below ground: the imperfectly buried corpse, the clogged sewer or drain. John Snow argued in 1849 that water polluted with fecal matter was the cause of cholera. He famously and graphically illustrated his theory by his removal of the handle of the Broad Street pump during a widely publicized outbreak linked to a well in St. James in 1854, thus intensifying public concern about hidden dangers below the surface of the city. The metaphor of palimpsestic depth so often used in this period's descriptions of urban space may be in part due to this shift—certainly it is evident in this excerpt, wherein human "refuse and scum" "boil up" and flow over the good, decent aboveground community.[5]

Once again, sanitarians took up the pen in reply, defending Palmerston. A caustic response in tract form (1853) reprinted sanitary advice given in letters in the *Times*, with a direct response to Buchanan in the introduction and conclusion:

> There are many persons who think they render the greatest homage to the Supreme Ruler, by contemplating the cholera and other epidemics as ministers of the Divine vengeance. . . . It is much to be lamented that inquiries into the physical causes of cholera have been rather deprecated than encouraged, from the impression that investigations of this nature were wanting in that humility and prostration which are appropriate to the visitation. ("The Laws of Cholera" 3–4)

The author concludes that "It is quite out of the question to get at the rationale of this epidemic by a sermon, or to stay its virulence by a Scotch fast or a popish mass. Religion is honoured when it is presented in harmony with nature, it is profaned when it is employed to secure immunity from the effects of violating her laws" ("The Laws of Cholera" 78–79). The writer here is on safe English grounds, and can afford to lump "Scotch fasts" and "popish masses" together. Religion generally is implicated, however, in the reference to "sermons," unmediated by an adjective.

THE ST. JAMES'S EPIDEMIC AND THE CRISIS OF INTERPRETATION

The confidence of the sanitarians was about to be badly shaken, however, by the cholera's sudden and horrifying volte-face in its preferred path. In 1854, the cholera returned. After a brief and inconclusive attack on its usual haunts, it broke out with unparalleled fury in the hitherto healthy—and wealthy—parish of St. James's, while the usually hardest hit areas were left relatively untouched.[6] Current concepts of sanitation and health were simply inadequate to engage this turn of events; the conceptual difficulties involved are perhaps best illustrated by the fact that by the fourth epidemic a decade later, this radical deviation from the norm was overlooked. At the time, however, its impact was profound. The 1855 *Report on the Cholera Outbreak in the Parish of St. James, Westminster, During the Autumn of 1854* suggests the difficulties of explaining the epidemic to the shocked inhabitants of St. James's; the report, in fact, is careful to impress upon its readers that there just *is* no way to make sense of it:

> There yet remain several characteristics of this visitation, which may here be noticed, as tending either to associate it with or distinguish it from other less severe and sudden outbreaks of the disease . . . [it did not stick to its old haunts, it was eccentric as usual in localization, preferring one side of the street to another]. Some narrow streets and courts suffered severely; others nearly or quite escaped, as Tyler's, Great Crown and Walker's Courts; whilst wide streets, as Broad Street itself, were heavily visited. . . . A want of cleanliness in streets or houses was by no means a constant accompaniment of the disease. Some houses in the midst of others affected escaped, without any favourable sanitary condition. (25–26)

Deaths are broken down by gender and occupation; tailors and bakers are noted as hardest hit, but the committee understandably didn't quite know what to do with this statistic, tentatively concluding (probably correctly) that perhaps this distribution emerged simply because mostly tailors and bakers lived there.

Other materials included suggest that one way in which local residents reconciled their perception of their district with their perception of cholera was by concluding that it either wasn't cholera at all, but something else, or that cholera, in their own case, proceeded from a unique environmental cause. The *Report* spends an extensive amount of space rebutting the argument that pest-fields underlying part of the parish, (that is, cemeteries dating from the time of the plague, dedicated by the then-owner of those lands, Lord Craven, to the interment of victims) had somehow generated the 1854 epidemic: "it has often been alleged that in some way or other the remains of decomposing animal matter, or indeed the plague matter itself, lying in the soil of this district, are chargeable with the great mortality from Cholera near it. Popular opinion has even gone so far as to maintain that the disease of last autumn was not Cholera, but a direful kind of black fever" (46). The report argues against this interpretation—why, after all, was St. James's spared in the previous two epidemics, when the plague matter was younger and therefore more potentially injurious? Still, the detailed attention given to the topic suggests a widespread currency.

In short, the public, at least in St. James's, was highly invested in retaining its notion of the cholera as a lower-class filth disease. The majority of victims in St. James's were respectable working class—often the same class as victims elsewhere. However, the general character of, say, St. Giles, a neighboring parish famous for its Irish slums, was sufficiently wretched to assimilate even a respectable tailor with the cholera to the general image of the inhabitants of the district as vicious and immoral. St. James's tailors, however, were not to be tarred with any such brush, as such would have affected the general image of the upper- and upper-middle-class community that inhabited the most important parts of the parish. John Snow's dramatic removal of the Broad Street pump handle in November of 1854, whereby he demonstrated his theory that the disease was spread through water contaminated with sewage, gave the report an "out." The report itself was generally favorable to Snow's interpretation (71); after all, the notion that one was being poisoned by the refuse of the adjacent poor was more tenable than being identified with them.

However, acceptance of Snow involved acceptance of two remarkable corollaries: one, that moral environmentalism was mistaken; two, that respectable and unrespectable society were not "two nations," but one, clearly united in body, if not in spirit. (Indeed, even as early as 1850, Charles Kingsley would point out the vulnerability of the upper classes to the disease of the lower through contagion in such tracts as *Cheap Clothes and Nasty*, in which sweated and starving tailors spread disease to their patrons through the clothing they sew. In the later general acceptance of germ theory, around the early '90s, one sees many references to the "socialism of the microbe" as a great leveler of humanity.[7]) Naturally, the clergy triumphantly rang the changes on the theme of national unity. Prominent evangelical clergyman Henry Venn Elliott points out in a published sermon addressed to the middle classes that

> familiarity with the scourge in a milder form took off the terror, till the disease, whether endemic or epidemic, came to be regarded as one which might, to a considerable extent, be provided against by public and private precautions. Cleanliness . . . and an early application of medicine and medical skill . . . were supposed to be specifics against the contagion. And to a certain extent there is some truth in these views; and it is thus that God enforces on us, by his great and invariable laws of health, the necessity of attention to these sanitary measures. But, pushing that truth too far, men began to map out the geographical boundaries of the malady. . . . Then the selfishness of our nature, leaving the poor in their disease or in their danger to pay the penalty of their localities, was heard to congratulate itself on the comparative safety of its better situations. . . . And then it was . . . that the cholera at one leap passed from the squalid abodes of poverty into the houses which were rejoicing in their comforts, and the streets which were high and clean. No districts, I hear, have suffered more from the cholera than certain parts of the parish of St. James's, and in certain vicinities of Oxford-street and Soho-square. . . . These events put an end to the fancied and selfish security of the healthier parts of London. (9–11)

Elliott wisely eschews the naming of a specific sin, keeping safely to the topic of the united community, but does point out that God visited the armies with cholera in the Baltic at the same time, to humble the nation and teach a lesson: "I confess I trembled when I read at the beginning of the war the arrogant and vaunting language of the public press. I feared it might be a mirror of the national mind" (24). Again, the press is seen as the public expression of sinfulness, and as the representative of national consciousness. The Reverend John Davies, Canon of Durham, reflects on the same topic in a sermon-cum-sixpennny tract: "In the movements and visitations of this scourge of God, as it may be justly called. . . . It's mode of attack is equally secret, unaccountable, capricious . . . [it attacks] persons of every age and sex, and habit of life" (5). He concludes, "That the calamity was punitive—that it was designed to mark God's displeasure with us for our sins individual and collective, may be justly argued from the general connection, which is observed and authoritatively declared to subsist between wickedness and suffering even in this life, as it bears upon the condition of nations and smaller communities" (11). This suffering, he argues, was obviously intended by God "to bring us to repentance and reformation, and thus ultimately to secure our happiness and well being throughout eternity," but he acknowledges that the specific lessons to be drawn are a bit murkier, and are hotly debated:

> To what extent, and in what respect the calamity, so fatal to the life of so many . . . is to be regarded in a special manner as a judgement of God upon us, has been made matter of frequent observation and discussion. Of the general fact there can be no question that when a kingdom, a nation, or a smaller community has sunk to a certain point of moral degradation . . . they are frequently visited in this capacity. . . . It is rarely safe for us, however, to fix, with absolute determination upon the peculiar forms of impiety and ungodliness, which have called forth these outpourings of divine anger. It is enough for us to know, and it is right that we should feel, that gross or wanton unfaithfulness to God in principle or practice on the part of nations or collective bodies of men, is a usual precursor of some marked and severe penal infliction. (11–13)

Once again, the author struggles to define the group that is culpable without specifying what, precisely, the sin is, and indeed, he suggests that it would be dangerous to attempt it. He also tries to skirt the dispute with sanitarians, who often argued that any discussion of a special judgment or "special providence" was a denial of the fixed laws of nature's cleanliness that sanitary nuisances violated. The violation of these fixed laws, many medics and sanitarians argued, resulted in epidemic disease. This might be a sin, but it was hardly one calling down a special judgment; in fact, some argued, the very notion of a special judgment invalidated the notion of general providence, or of a science that would allow humans to know nature and live in accordance with it. Davies cautions, "In thus recognizing the hand of God in these awful providential visitations, we do not, as is sometimes alleged, intend for a moment to deny the existence of general and fixed laws, nor the spontaneous action of physical and secondary causes. The laws of nature . . . are . . . the creatures of an omnipotent will" (11–13).

Regarding the critique of religious attitudes toward cholera by sanitarians, he is finally dismissive:

> I do not now enter into the futile—futile, I mean, so far as it relates to its moral and religious aspect—and unanswerable question, how far local and physical agencies have been concerned in this recent visitation, or into the equally unanswerable question, what may be the special, national, or personal sins, which have called it forth out of the dread treasury of God's displeasure. It is enough for us to know that it was an instrument of his chastisement and reproof of us, and that it was designed to lead us to repentance. (24)

In this argument, he simply subsumes medical authority under religious authority—"physical and secondary causes" are simply the tools God uses; the job of understanding those tools is of secondary importance to the interpretation of

God's will. Specific human actions are less significant in this sermon than in some others; one need not dwell on the "futile" and "unanswerable" question of the nature of the sin. In fact, he makes it seem almost irreligious to enquire. The move of incorporating "sanitary laws" or "secondary causes" into divine action is more and more frequently used throughout the period, but it rarely seems to be an entirely comfortable compromise, and seems more to be a way of avoiding a debilitating and inconclusive struggle.

Meanwhile, the official death rates of around fifty percent and admissions of confoundment like the 1854 St. James's *Report on the Cholera Outbreak* invited attack from the margins of the medical profession, such as from the increasing numbers of homeopathic practitioners, who sensed that the time was ripe for an attack on the "hidebound institution" of allopathy, or traditional medicine. Homeopaths debated approaching Parliament with a petition to abolish allopathy in the Boards of Health, and were guardedly courteous to the clergy, who seemed like possible allies. By the 1840s, homeopaths had become very popular in Britain, and by the late 1840s were recognized as a threat by the traditional medical profession, who began to engage in systematic institutional harassment of those espousing such tenets.[8] James John Garth Wilkinson, noted homeopath and scholar, makes an appeal to both public and clergy in the introduction to his 1854 book on homeopathy:

> There cannot be a doubt that sin is the effectual caller of all misery, and that the cholera is a consequence of our sins. These sins, however, are of many kinds, and it is not about those which have a simply religious bearing that I am going to speak. Physical and medical sins, acknowledged as such in the sight of God also, are those which I shall try to bring home to you, in order that their special repentance, and a regeneration thereafter, may be ensured. Other repentances are urged by other appointed voices, and to them also let us respond, Amen. (1)

Having offered this guarded nod to the clergy, while still staking out a specifically "physical and medical" territory as separate from the spiritual realm, he immediately proceeds to an attack on traditional medicine:

> The British nation, like every other in Christendom, contains within it many solid and compact organizations which have come from old times, and which have well-nigh all power in several great departments of action and thought. Among these are the professions, medical, clerical, legal, and many others. Huge social fortresses, they stand above the interests of individual houses, nominally for protection and defence. Yet there is not one of them but supports a continual siege against its own times and peoples; and what is termed reform is always accompanied by the razing of some part of their

outworks, or of the very citadels themselves. . . . The medical profession, with its black innumerable donjons, is at present brought, by the benignant pestilence, into clear opposition with the interests of man. (1–2)

So instead of a calling to spiritual repentance, the cholera becomes a calling to scientific, social, and professional reform. He concludes that the "medical profession, as such, is confessedly powerless in the presence of cholera" and that, further, "Medical science itself has the disease in its most virulent form. Not a remedy keeps upon its irritable stomach from day to day. . . . Convulsed and blue-cold, half death and half physic, it chatters out its horrible statistics. In place of a fountain of health, it is, in science, the focus and epitome of the pestilence of the time" (3). The profession, here, becomes the source of cholera itself. Wilkinson's vision of the medical profession may seem absurdly monolithic for such a young and vexed professional group; however, allopathy was powerful enough to preserve a dignified silence in the face of such accusations, at least at the book and pamphlet level, if not within the more intimate venues of professional journals.

The preceding passage sees medicine (at least traditional medicine) as a coherent institution, with some pretensions to public service, but these "social fortresses" of professional exclusion are now at war with the society they historically have served. Cholera, which so often operates as a metaphor for systemic national corruption, has got hold of medicine itself, "convulsed and blue-cold . . . chattering out its horrible statistics"—so that medicine and the sanitarians, who were then still largely those producing the horrible statistics, are linked. As in the church's rhetoric and in radical working-class rhetoric, cholera is not only something that enables professional control of public and private life, it is a product and symptom of institutional and social irresponsibility. Homeopathic writers complained of being kept out of the press—not only professional venues like the *Lancet*, but the *Times* as well. Regardless of their marginality in the profession, however, they enjoyed an enduring popularity with patients, and boasted, probably accurately, a much lower death rate than regular practitioners, whose favorite remedies for cholera still included calomel (mercury) and bleeding.

Other rumblings of discontent within the profession came from traditionally allopathic practitioners who were concerned with the difficulties of negotiating between the heroic, altruistic, and public-spirited vision of medicine as a profession and the traditional business orientation of the "leech." Physician John Grove averred that "Until our profession, as a whole, shall have cast off the trammels of trade, it will neither obtain the merit it deserves, nor secure the esteem of which it stands in need, because the people, generally speaking, look to the physic, not to the physician's talent, as that which is to be paid for" (42). He also complained, in a lament that seems eerily familiar today, that doctors spent more time on their ledgers and business records than detailing cases and providing solid medical statistics (42–43). As historian Anne Digby points out, this altruism was largely enforced, rather than voluntary (253). Working-class friendly societies (similar to insurance cooperatives) organized consumers against a disorganized medical profession, members of which constantly undercut each other through competition. The New Poor Law created medical positions that young doctors were encouraged to take to build their careers, but whose pay was exploitative at best.

Parish Unions resented the money doctors asked for, often seeing them as taking advantage of the cholera panic. Under the "West London Union" section of "The Cholera" in the *City Press*, a Mr. Butcher objected to the appointment of two medical officers at an extra £10 per week for the cholera visitations, insisting that "Medical Officers might easily create a sensation to get £10 a-week. (Cries of 'oh-oh!')," in 1866 (6). The same year, a Poor Law Guardian stated that medical officers were practically on strike, neglecting to send in reports on cholera. Physician Robert Fowler, the district medical officer of the East London Union, responded, "The City Union Medical Officers require in this matter neither the recognition, nor the duty, nor the pay. But if the Court of Sewers demands the duty, the Medical Officers demand the pay. They cannot recognize the justice or morality of expecting from them that gratuitous patriotism which no other class of the community is supposed to contribute" ("Cholera in the City" 3). Making a living in the medical field was quite difficult, and the desire of privileged medics to preserve status differences retarded the development of professional unity that would have protected the economic interests of less privileged practitioners.[9]

HOW THE CRISIS RESOLVED: CHOLERA IN THE 1860s

On the whole, however, the triumph of critics of the "sanitary point of view" was short-lived. The challenge posed by the eruption of cholera in St. James's was insufficient to upset the perception of cholera as a poverty disease, and the increasing respect given to science as a truth discourse—as well as the number of clergy actively involved in sanitarian pursuits—eventually made it expedient for religious writers to admit the validity of "proximate causes." With the threat of disestablishment essentially past, and the advent of highly publicized doctrinal diversity spawned under the agency of John Henry Newman,[10] the ritualists, and others, the clergy's positions were more widely divergent than in the first epidemic and reflected more personal points of view about the nature of science, faith, fallen humanity, and so forth. Although some clergy were offended by the materialism of science, many more were supportive and often engaged in scientific pursuits themselves. By the fourth and last epidemic of the mid '60s, a Ladies' Sanitary Association tract places the sanitarian's discourse in the mouth of the clergy, and the opposing religious explanation is perceived to come from the ignorant "village" parishioners:

> It pained the Vicar's heart to see
> The pale and sickly faces,
> And know that suffering and disease
> Had made those ghastly traces.
>
> For none believed him when he spoke
> Of cause and of effect;
> It seemed so strange to hear him say
> 'Twas from their own neglect.
>
> Some had a notion it was *wrong*
> To trace out cause of ill;
> Submission was the Christian's part—
> Submission to God's will.
>
> (Ladies' Sanitary Association)

In this verse narrative—which continues at some length—the vicar carries out a sanitary siege on his backward parishioners, who insist that God is the source of epidemics, and that death and disease must be piously accepted. They are brought to recognize the truth when the vicar and his helpers fill in the wells and clean out the ponds, which contain "near ten feet of mire." Reverend William Dean Buckland's 1849 sermon on the Day of Thanksgiving after the epidemic is strongly sanitarian, though he still manages to blame the victims, saying it is mostly the vicious and intemperate who die, even if sometimes the good suffer along with the guilty (19). He then cites extensively from the Metropolitan Commissioner of Sewers *Reports* of 1849 and James Glaisher's report in particular, in an appendix at the back of the published sermon, using the sanitary discourse as a form of support for the primary matter of the sermon.[11]

On the medical side, the same move toward conflation of the two discourses is evident. Dr. George Johnson, speaking to a missionary group, airily ridiculed the natives of India, without apparent understanding that the beliefs he ridiculed existed in living memory in his own country, and were considered mainstream:

Cholera they ["Hindoos"] believe to be caused by the direct agency of a deity, and not the result of avoidable physical causes. Without doubt, great judgement and caution are required in dealing with deep-seated hereditary superstitions and prejudices, but we may reasonably hope that the time is not far distant when the natives of India may learn that the only sure preventive of cholera is through cleanliness in their persons, their dwellings, their food, and above all in their drink. . . . Such teaching by degrees may do much to free them from those superstitions which hinder the general reception of Christianity. (26–27)

Here, sanitary views that in the late 1840s had been perceived as opposed to religious orthodoxy are seen as promoting it. By 1866, this view seems to be generally accepted. However, the Church of England continued, if not with the fast day, with at least the special cholera liturgy, with its rhetoric of self-accusation.[12]

In the 1866 liturgy, clergy are directed to pray, "we approach Thee under a deep sense of our sinfulness, and in awe of Thy Judgments which are abroad in the Pestilence that has now reached our shores. We desire to humble ourselves . . . confessing our iniquities which have justly provoked Thy wrath against us." I have only found a few published sermons on the topic of national guilt in this period, one of which is certainly worth quoting at length. The Reverend Hugh M'Neile, a scriptural literalist best known for his many published denunciations of Rome and for his Greek edition of the Gospel of Matthew, boldly attributes agency to God, and is, in the only example I have seen, bold in identifying the national sin:

it is plain, as plain as any conclusion of reason, that wars, famines, pestilences, whether on man or beast or both, commercial panics, social convulsions, are all God's personal actings in our world, through whatever second causes, or chains of events, they are introduced. These are not arbitrary unmeaning acts, unconnected with any moral government over man. On the contrary, they form an important part of that government, and are expressly declared to be punishments for sin. (8)

He quotes the prayer, and asks his audience to think about it; unlike several of the sermons from the 1850s, he insists on naming specific sins: "Now, supposing us to be sincere with God . . . we ought surely to have some distinct perception of what our sins are. How can we be sorry for them, how can we forsake them without knowing what they are? Search, therefore and see what sins you mean, when you join in this prayer. What share have you had personally in provoking God to send the cholera?" (8–9). He reasons that if his auditors have not sinned, they will be sinning by reciting the prayer: "If there be nothing, if you have not been knowingly and willfully violating any law of God, how can you take part in such a confession as this? Is it not mere flattery with your mouth?" (9). He also distinguishes between individual and national sin, noting that "it is by no means clear that the sins of private individuals as such, are the only or even the chief cause of *national* calamities. . . . For such persons as individuals there remains an eternity" (9). A nation, however, "*as a nation*, has no eternity to spend. It is a temporal thing. Temporal prosperity is its glory, its heaven, its only heaven. Temporal calamity is its punishment, the only punishment it is capable of. National punishments, as described in the word of God, are destructive wars, pestilences, famines and such like, and they are expressly declared to be incurred and deserved by national sins" (9–10). Having sorted out that cholera is a punishment for national rather than individual sin, he proceeds directly to the stickiest of wickets: "What are *national* sins? Do they consist of the aggregate of the sins of the individuals composing the nation? This is the common idea, but it is attended with no small difficulty and embarrassment. For, consider. Is every sin of every individual a national sin? This will scarcely be pretended" (10–11). Murder, he points out, is not a national sin, because even though it takes place within a nation, the feeling of the nation is against it. Nations sin, then, only as nations act: "BY THEIR RULERS. . . . England acts by her Parliament" (11). A national sin must be committed by national authority through Parliamentary action. The specific national sin in question, it turns out, is the toleration of a Catholic seminary, endowed with state funding through Parliament, in contrariety to the stipulations against "idolatry" of the Church of England (11). This sermon deviates from those of previous epidemics in some important ways. Most importantly, it does not concern itself with establishing a connection between nation and individual; although it begins by insisting on the identification of individual guilt, it becomes a political critique of leadership, having little to do with individual repentance. It also assumes a model of representative government, in which state is not separate from nation. M'Neile was at the extreme conservative fringe of the Anglican church in this period, yet he was not completely isolated; he was part of a then-important group of religious thinkers at Albury, where he was rector when this was written.

Still, it is probable there were not many sermons like this in 1866—certainly, if there were, they were not being printed as tracts. At least one anonymous critic, however, took the prayer seriously enough to speak out against it, charging it with "perversity"—"a national sin it surely must be, to speak ill of God in public prayer" ("A Protest," 6). The prayer, the author argues, charges God with cruelty, denies the power of science, blames the sufferers, makes them afraid (which itself causes cholera), and keeps people from helping the stricken for fear that they are working against the will of god. Blaming the victims is cruel, because "three things are known to all. First, that there . . . is as much sin in the rich West End of London as in the poor East and South. Secondly, that the rich will escape, or nearly quite escape, the Cholera. Thirdly, that only particular districts have suffered, and that many of those who have suffered and died, and who will suffer and die, have been and will be little children of the poor" ("A Protest" 4). The writer further charges that not a single clergyman in England will publicly admit to believing such things, implying that the prayer is simply outdated. The experience of smaller, classed groups is elevated as a defining characteristic of the epidemic and the community's experience of it; the nation's unity in suffering is exposed as false and disingenuous.

The Reverend Gordon Calthrop, editor of the *Home Visitor* magazine, took a swing at this problem in a sermon published in 1865. On the subject of "national judgments," he notes, his parishioners had begun the prior Sunday "to use a form of prayer in which we confessed our sins" and asked to be spared the cholera that has devastated other countries (9). This, he suggests, may strike some as old-fashioned: "Now it cannot be unknown to you . . . that . . . the utterance of the pulpit [on this topic] will be decidedly at variance with the prevailing spirit of the age. The God of a large and influential section of our fellow-countrymen is NATURAL LAW" (9–10). He hedges his bets by implying that the populace has failed in its duties to God, which include observance of sanitary laws (15), and then offers a long justification for why such an intervention would be "in character." He implies that most people will be incredulous, but urges parishioners to consider:

> it is a likely thing that God should occasionally make himself felt . . . in the history of a nation . . . experience tells us that no condition is so adverse to the growth and development of the spiritual life, as that in which we enjoy long-continued, unbroken prosperity and success. Now what is true of individuals is also true of that aggregate of individuals, which we call a nation . . . knowing what we do about the love of God, and his care . . . we should *expect* Him, when dealing with men in their corporate capacity as peoples, to make Himself felt, on occasion, by some special and intelligible interposition. (10–11)

Calthorp manages to make the cholera sound like quite a favor, a mark of God's personal fondness for a Britain already richly showered with his blessings. (This is perhaps unintentionally opposed to earlier explanations that saw the cholera logically as a sign of God's displeasure precisely because it was one of many simultaneous tribulations.) However, by this time, the "nation as aggregate" definition, though still having some currency, was yielding to a more sophisticated model of representation such as M'Neile's.

Curate Henry Whitehead, in his pamphlet "The Cholera in Berwick Street" (which was not a sermon, but a journalistic account of his experiences that supported Snow's explanation for the St. James's outbreak), uses the language of natural law and comments that "surely it is a sin, a national sin, that the poor should be condemned to live as they do" (10). Some disagreement with this position is evident in the sermon published by the incumbent of St.

Luke's, Reverend Samuel Arnott, who recommends Whitehead's forthcoming pamphlet to the public, but, without commenting directly on Whitehead's doctrine, insists that Divine Judgment is not inconsistent with general providence (7). For Arnott, the cholera is clearly a judgment, though he remarks that "I would not for a moment suppose, that our District has been selected as a place of Divine judgment, because the sins of the inhabitants are more aggravated . . . from whatever cause, the disease scarcely passed beyond Little Pulteney Street" (9), and, he argues, the people on the other side of Little Pulteney Street are certainly no better than they are on his side. He notes that the innocent suffer with the guilty, but charges his parish generally with infidelity and nonobservance of the Sabbath, and devotes a page detailing the titles of books and pamphlets—with prices and locations to purchase—that he feels his parishioners should acquire to read on Sundays (16).

In any case, the official liturgy may well have been viewed by many as an empty form by then, a kind of statement legitimated by tradition that did not really imply what it so clearly said. Medics did not bother to publicly challenge the clergy in this period, which may suggest that either the clergy were not generally taking a firm cholera-is-punishment position, or that those few who did were not taken as mainstream. By this time, religion—the vicar, the missionaries—was put into the service of conveying truth to the public, and that truth was determined not only by church interpretations of doctrine but by medical interpretations of scientific study. Clergy became the secular go-between for the oracular scientist and the public—and science was recuperated as the expression and servant of Divine Will. Though a moral failing was still implied in the 1860s, it was the failing of a "civilized" society to keep itself clean. It was not, generally, that the poor are seen as any more morally upstanding than earlier, but that the task of society itself was perceived to be overseeing and disciplining the bodies of the poor. Sin was punished, in a largely mechanical universe, by the immutable laws of Nature, set in motion by God perhaps, but not vitally and intimately connected with individual acts of divine will.

The early medical vision isolated the individual body. One was culpable for specifically physical sins, which were one's own, not shared. Although sanitarian moral environmentalism defined communities around their collective ordure, the actual medical discourse of the case study located the causes of cholera in individual habits. Although temperance was an overlapping concern with the clergy, medical science did not rhetorically link intemperance to ungodliness; intemperance was bad because it upset the homeostatic balance of the body. It involved reckless expenditures of energy, but, more crucially, it involved taking in too much, which would then have to be drained, through venesection, blistering, and so forth. The care of the self in the first half of the century involved a narrow moderation and accounting of intake; it did not involve absolute self-denial, which was figured as a different kind of imbalance or intemperance. The church's rhetoric, with its emphasis on self-denial (e.g., fasting), was directly at odds with this vision of the body. Further, the religious response to emergency involved a heightening of spiritual and emotional activity, whereas medical science prescribed calm and a more absolute adherence to homeostasis. To some clergy, it also seemed blasphemous to suggest that sanitation and medical care of the self could redeem one from the results of what they considered part of our fallen nature.

But even more importantly, the mid-century began to see the emergence of a modern liberal society. This society depended on the establishment of institutionalized expert biopolitical knowledges, or *savoirs*, (for example, the sanitary movement and its materialization in public health legislation) for the formation of the liberal subject, capable of self-regulation in the service of the modern state.[13] Medicine was one of the privileged systems of expertise by which the social, as a domain of knowledge and control, was constituted. This process, crucial in the 1860s discussion of fitness for the franchise in the expanding electorate, depended both on the benevolent surveillance of the populace by experts in the service of the state, and on the didactic discourse of those experts, which hailed workers through a rhetoric of patriotic communitarianism and membership in a healthy social body.

Whereas in 1831, members' speeches identify the elimination of violent mob activity as a primary goal, and the promotion of economically desirable activity as a secondary goal of reform, speeches in the '60s imply a much more complex set of goals for working-class behavior, as well as the elimination, rather than simple control, of pauperism. Many of these goals were explicitly to be reached through sanitary strategies (such as better housing, cleanliness, and the elimination of food adulteration), and these, in turn, were explicitly linked to the franchise. Thus, a shared national identity emerged in the context of a radically (medically) connected social body, in which all of the constituent parts had the ability to affect one another—or, conversely, had no ability *not* to. Public health was a technology for managing the health of this social body, which was intimately connected to morality and therefore socialization.

For the church to maintain its position as "speaker for the nation," it had to do two things: first, extend its audience beyond the middle classes to tradespeople, workers, and the poor (as the ritualists attempted to do throughout the '50s and '60s); and, second, align itself with the expert knowledges of political economy and public health. In this way, the church could retain some of its authority at the parish level, as mediator between the people and the state, especially as medical relief was coordinated through the parish authorities. On the other hand, the rhetoric of nationhood was largely absent from medical writing through the earlier epidemics. As previously noted, medical discourse provided ways to talk about the individual body and about sanitary topography, yet about the activity of human community, it was silent. However, in the fourth epidemic, about the time the church drops this issue, medical discourse finds a way to make central "English" identity, and that is within the discourse of racial biology. I would argue that the change is partially in the overall medical view of humanity and the body—defined in part by a new attention to racial traits and the evolutionary model, as we shall see more clearly in later chapters.

The rhetoric of nationhood, with its complex negotiation of the relationship of the individual to the larger group, intersected with the discourses surrounding the cholera with particular urgency, becoming a site upon which authority and identity were constructed and contested. Biopolitical *savoirs* crucial to the centralization and formation of the liberal state and those subjected to it insured that, to retain its centrality as a national symbol, the church had to appropriate to itself an interest in those knowledges and claim a space within their practice. By the end of the period, the domains of the body and soul were, at least in this respect, rendered both fully disaggregated and seamlessly complementary.

3

A Suffering Nation

Responses of the Poor and Radicals to the Cholera

HOMI BHABHA HAS SAID that the rhetoric of "nation" performs a double gesture, both constituting the people as an audience for a didactic discourse of nation and as a subject which speaks that discourse (298–300). In 1832, political reform constituted the subject of that discourse in a new way, suggesting the possibility that a national subject with the simple qualification of respectability (defined as inhabiting property worth rents of £10 per annum) might define himself as such through the exercise of the franchise.[1] It identified the object of that discourse, however, as two divergent groups: one, educable, respectable, capable of evolving into a responsible electorate; the other, an aggregate of humanity, reduced to a merely physical subjectivity, from whom very little could be expected but docile obedience to the interests of the electorate and therefore the nation with which they were to identify.[2] That category was further subdivided into the working poor and, finally, the pauper class, which were truly the "heathens" and "aliens" within their own community. In short, the oscillation between those positions—as subject and object of national discourse—at the margins of economic entitlement where the cholera threat was perceived to reside was what the church (and the medical profession) had to address, in order to define itself as teacher/speaker for the nation. It is precisely this oscillation, as well, that working-class radicals targeted to expose the ideological inconsistencies of the authorities' position.

The classes that sanitarians and clergy intended to represent and control had their own interpretations of the cholera epidemics, conspicuously absent from the official narratives of the disease. As authorities wrangled over definitions of cholera, its causes, treatment, and prophylaxis, the classes most largely and publicly victimized by cholera were also engaged in the process of interpretation. Their narratives are not as accessible as those of officialdom, but some aspects are recoverable. The readings that we can recapture from personal histories, broadsheets, radical newspapers, and so forth, suggest that many among the working classes saw the cholera in terms of negative social control, providing an opportunity for the upper classes to seize working-class rights, voices, and even bodies.

CHOLERA, NATION, AND CLASS: 1832

The first epidemic immediately was inscribed within narratives of class struggle. The rhetorical tactics used were various, but break down into the following: denial of the existence of cholera and accusations of jobbery and conspiracy against the poor; redefinition of cholera as a political rather than a medical problem; narratives of class genocide (based loosely on popular understandings of Malthus and associated with the census); and body-snatcher narratives, in which the cholera might or might not be real but provided a pretext for the literal appropriation of the bodies of the poor, who might not be actually dead at the time of being "burked." In all of these responses, there was a commonality of perception that the surveillance and regulation of the bodies of the poor amounted to an attempt to actually seize control of those bodies, most graphically illustrated by the forced removal and containment of the ill in hastily built cholera hospitals. Many simply disbelieved in the existence of cholera.[3] Rioting and violence against medics and some clergy gives evidence that some of these sentiments extended beyond the few who have left published records of their views.[4]

This distrust led to parodic counter-narratives, such as the folk prescription that drinking alcohol would keep the cholera away (as opposed to the widely disseminated statements of medics and clergy that drinking would cause the cholera), or the more politically conscious declaration by labor organizations of feast days in opposition to the public fast declared by Parliament and the Church of England.[5] Such gestures dramatized the opposing physical circumstances in which rich and poor lived. These also were powerful fragmenting narratives, asserting, in the face of the tales of national unity advanced by the authorities, a clear difference in the lived experience of classes who did not feel part of a national shared experience.

Some of this dialogue was articulated in the radical press and broadsheets. Some radicals interpreted the cholera as a red herring designed to get the attention of the public off reform:

> They tell such tales our hearts to fear
> Of Cholera raging here and there,
> But bread, pudding, and good cheer,
> Will drive the Cholera Morbus . . . //
>
> But Reformers will not be deceived,
> For by them it is all agreed
> That one and all we shall be freed,
> In spite of the Cholera Morbus.
>
> (Broadsheet, "A New Song")

This ballad, addressed to "Britons," evokes a different kind of national unity than that envisioned by the church liturgy—a national unity that certainly excludes antireformers, and the doctors and clergy as well, to the extent that they are seen as allies of the elite. In Ely, for example, notices saying "No cholera at Ely / The Parsons Liars / And Doctors Pickpockets" were pasted over handbills distributed by the Board of Health (in Holmes 32–33). Radical press and labor organizations emphasized the absurdity of the solutions proposed by the upper classes for an audience in very different circumstances. Radical printer and activist Henry Hetherington of *The Poor Man's Guardian*—who himself died of cholera in 1849 (Durey 195)—ridiculed the notion of the general fast day through several issues, beginning on February 11, 1832, "a *general fast* is all very fair; for God knows that as yet the fasting has been *partial* enough . . . if not merely fasting but if the most abject want be any propitiation for the evil, never would CHOLERA MORBUS have made its appearance among us!" (1). Hetherington related the fast to the issue of national unity:

> we can come to no other conclusion than that you, the poor and lower classes, are not those to whom the Proclamation is addressed . . . the language is "we, and our people"; and "people" we know, are "contradistinguished from the mob and the populace"—at the most, including the £10 householders; nor is it probable that our government would consider it at all likely that an Almighty God could condescend to acknowledge [the poor]. (274)

Besides, he argues, whatever sins there may be, "deserving 'heavy judgements,' there is, again, no reason you should adopt *them*: you have not murdered, in cold blood, your Bristol and Nottingham fellow creatures—you do not idly revel in luxuries while your slaving brethren are wanting necessaries!" (274). He closes by assuring his readers that they can also hardly expect, under such circumstances, to be the 'loving subjects' designated in the proclamation. The language of reform is used explicitly to reinforce the schism between the class to whom it is addressed and the government that "hails" them, but that does not consider them to be worthy of direct political representations, as such people do not meet the minimal financial qualification for the franchise even under the new Reform Bill. He especially targets the contradictions between medical and clerical approaches as an argumentative tool: "Bye the bye, the *Figaro in London* shrewdly remarks upon the inconsistency of providing, as a remedy for the disease, the very condition which 'the faculty' have determined, most invites the attack; viz., the *want of proper food*" (Hetherington 1).

Even the mainstream press agreed in lampooning the class blindness of such a prescription. *Punch*, in a tart blurb entitled "Advice Gratis," published a satirical notice from the "college of Physicians"—"Everyone is to live extremely well [to avoid cholera]. . . . All persons crowded together in small ill-ventilated houses are recommended to take at once more commodious apartments and those individuals who are insufficiently clothed must give orders forthwith to their tailors" (207). Apparently, some employers believed that, for some, the fast days could become a day of freedom instead of "self-abasement." One broadsheet from Braintree states that a public fast would be impious and unlawful and that factories would not close. However, it is reluctantly conceded that if hands *really* were to make it a religious observance and not a holiday, they might have the day off (Broadsheet, Place Collection).[6]

The popular ballad "A New Song on the Cholera Morbus," printed as a broadsheet, runs the gamut of radical beliefs and rumors about cholera (Broadsheet, "A New Song"). First questioning the reality of cholera, the verses identify "the Cholera Morbus" with inequities in living conditions, and suggest jobbery:

> In every street as you pass by
> Take care, they say, or you will die
> While others cry "It's all my eye,"
> There is no Cholera Morbus.
>
> If the Cholera Morbus should come here,
> The best of clothes you then must wear,
> Eat and drink the best, then never fear,
> You will get no Cholera Morbus,
>
> . . . Some people say it was a puff,
> It was done to raise the doctor's stuff
> And there has now been near enough
> About the Cholera Morbus.

The verses don't spare the church or medics:

> . . . If you should drink either beer or gin
> Or any liquor, what a sin.
> You would have the Cholera Morbus.

> . . . In Parliament of late did pass
> A motion for a general Fast,
> And if it very long should last
> It may bring the Cholera Morbus.

The ballad then shifts to explicitly political and economic troubles, advocating reform:

> This nation long has troubles borne,
> The people has been left forlorn,
> It was reported that the Reform
> Had caught the Cholera Morbus.

> . . . But I'm not afraid, says Royal WILL
> I must watch the Tories, and the Bill,
> And I'll send the villains for to dwell,
> Where they'll get the Cholera Morbus.

> . . . It is my opinion, as a man,
> That trade as [*sic*] long been at a stand,
> There's thousands starving through the land
> And that's the Cholera Morbus.

> Some live in luxury, some deplore,
> And if the rich don't help the poor
> When the D—gets them to his door,
> They have the Cholera Morbus.

> Pray don't be frightened great or small,
> The Cholera won't come here at all.
> If it does, it will the Tories call,
> Indeed the Cholera Morbus.

The nation that long has troubles born is either identical with or unable to assist the unitary group of "people" that "has been left forlorn." It seems it is the Parliament (at least the Tory contingent) which is to blame, thus separating state from nation, but identifying people with nation (and king) against state. The religious lesson to be taken, the ballad suggests, is that the uncharitable rich are the sinners and that the cholera will be their punishment. The cholera—which may or may not exist as a real disease—functions at several metaphorical levels here: as poverty, sin, political corruption, and economic problems. The fungibility of the metaphor—its overdetermined nature and simultaneous fluidity—suggests that writers were dealing with a kind of mytheme, or mythological building block, at the level of "nation" or "patriotism"; it was up for grabs, explaining so many problems it was available to almost any discourse. The balladeer satirizes this fluidity. The term "cholera" took on this connotative burden before the actual disease arrived in England. Upon its arrival, of course, actual illness and deaths forestalled the absolute free play of cholera as metaphor—cholera became something real, and quite particular. Yet, the disease retained the weight of its metaphoric associations with the nation's political, economic, and social health.

Another more subtle satire, also on broadsheet, reads, "Cholera Morbus! Any person supplying the Board of Health with a few cases of Asiatic Cholera will receive a liberal and substantial Reward. . . . Apply at the Commission Room, at any hour. No questions will be asked and *no mistake dreamt of*" (Broadsheet, "Cholera Morbus!"). It is signed "Aesculapius, Jun. and Co." Here the strong focus is on the suspicion of jobbery, with the emphasis on medical science as a business supported by the falsification of statistics at the public expense. This may be a middle-class satire, as tradespeople resented the quarantine restrictions initially imposed in the first epidemic. Almost certainly it was trade pressure that resulted in the quarto poster printed in Kidderminster in which ten "Medical Practitioners of the Town" affirmed that they had no cases of Cholera under their care and that "There is no such Disorder now existing in our town" (Broadsheet, "There Is No Such Disorder"). Small traders' antipathy for medical interventions into business are also evident in a quarto broadsheet that blames doctors, who, it is claimed, are the grocers' best customers, for forbidding the use of fruit and vegetables in order to guarantee themselves a supply of patients— this is the true cause of "Why is the Cholera Morbus raging in London?": "CHOLERA MORBUS. The Growers can prove, that not one Case of Cholera has taken place among the thousands of poor people they employ . . . who chiefly live upon that wholesome produce" (Broadsheet, "Cholera Humbug"). But accusations of jobbery were frequent also in the radical press, and may well have reflected the well-established cynicism the poor had about the motives of doctors and the well-to-do in general. A letter to the *Poor Man's Guardian* in 1832 and the editorial response are illustrative: "Sir,—I beg leave to invite your attention to a report . . . that the physicians appointed by the Board of Health, are to have £20 (or guineas) per diem. If this is true, which *you* can perhaps ascertain, is it not an additional proof that the Cholera is as complete a JOB as most things in this country are." The letter is immediately followed by the response that the editor does not know how much the "small fry" or doctors subordinated to the chief inspector make, but "We will undertake, however, to promise that the Cholera will remain in this country as long as the pay lasts" (295).[7]

Radicals also targeted the lack of charity displayed by the wealthy with heavy irony, implying that the recognition of the needs of the working classes should not be considered charity by other members of the national body, but simple recompense for labor, and, more obliquely, attacking the lack of Christian "charity" or religious tolerance evoked by the reference to the body metaphor in I Corinthians 12:12 in sermons on church and national unity. Of course, charity had another popular meaning, and it is this meaning that working-class radicals mobilized against the church's discourse of unity in sin and guilt; where, they asked, was that material charity that is the bond of recognition between the wealthy and poor in times of crisis? And where was the unity of charity in a nation divided against itself on the basis of the £10 qualification? Many letters from readers in radical publications duplicate this tone, and several working-class organizations declared a "general feast" to be celebrated on the fast day, in which food would be distributed free to the poor.

In a partial inversion of the existing dynamic, radicals acknowledged cholera as a filth disease (as they also often sided with temperance), but blamed the condition of the poor upon the wealthy: "It is a disease born of that poverty and wretchedness which are occasioned by the wealth and luxury of the few to whom only the constitution belongs. . . . But let our masters tremble in their palaces,—let them know that this *disease* is a retaliating scourge, and will sting the hands of those who inflict it . . . the beggar who dies at the door of the palace, poisons the air which circulates through it" (*Poor Man's Guardian* 281). The writer remarks that the cholera is fostered by trade, taking a contagionist position against the explicit anticontagionism of the government and adding to it the sanitary position that the conditions of poverty contributed to the disease:[8] "They have allowed their commerce to communicate the infection, nor have they attempted to relieve or improve that miserable condition of the poor which . . . actually generates the contagion:— they talked, to be sure, of doing something, *out of charity* . . . but, having consoled themselves that the rich have nothing to fear, their '*charity*' became extinct" (*Poor Man's Guardian* 281).

WORKERS, THE POOR, AND THEIR
REACTION TO MEDICAL INTERVENTION

Of course, it is difficult to say how many working-class and/or poor people would have shared this attitude, but what we do know something about is their reaction to the actions of the medical profession. Although very little of the non-organized working-class reaction enters "official" accounts of the cholera, one can recover a good deal from memoirs and local newspapers, "reading between the lines." It is evident that there was much resistance to the seizure of bodies, to early burial, and the like. Rioting was widespread, as was destruction of cholera carts and the hospitals. Medics were often attacked. Some may have believed that cholera was a scheme to get rid of the surplus population that had been identified by the census of 1831:[9] "The people, they [poor people] assert, have been numbered and classified for the purpose of selecting the most populous districts wherein this new disorder might be introduced," medic Thomas Doherty writes in 1832 (in Morris 98–99). Hospitals, he adds, were viewed simply as jobbery, "and a means of removing the poor sick from the sight of their friends so that they may more conveniently be anatomised by the doctors" (in Morris 98–99). Similar fears were expressed all over Europe. François Delaporte notes that Parisians feared that the government and the doctors were poisoning them, whereas hygienists there fueled the fears of the populace by publicly stating that pestilence was Nature's answer to overpopulation (51–52).

But the majority of Britons were more concerned with the seizure of the bodies by anatomists than with poisoning. Feeding this panic were the recent grave-robbing and murder trial of Burke and Hare, as well as Parliamentary deliberations on the "Dead Body Bill" or Anatomy Act, passed in 1832. The act, which provided that bodies of paupers not claimed within forty-eight hours by family members able to pay for interment would be available for dissection, was designed to relieve the lack of dissectable bodies that led to grave-robbing. It also had the effect of making the poor particularly vulnerable to the seizure of their bodies after death. It was unfortunately the case that there were a few doctors who were taking advantage of the seclusion of cholera patients in hospitals and hasty burials. One of the most dramatic occurrences resulted in the September 2nd Manchester cholera riot (Morris 110). John Hase[10] had brought his four-year-old grandson to the hospital, and was denied entry when he came to visit, being told that the child was convalescent. When next he came, he was told the child had died and been buried. He went with several friends and exhumed the body, and found that the child's corpse was headless. The bereaved grandfather carried the casket through the town, mustering a crowd later estimated at three thousand people, demanding justice. (Later inquiry revealed that a doctor—who left town precipitously during the riots and did not return—had bribed the nurse to allow him to carry off the head after the boy's death.) Doctors were pelted with stones and filth by crowds screaming the epithet "Burkers!" and several patients were "liberated" from the hospitals and carried triumphantly away. This is perhaps the most dramatic of many incidents, but the general attitude of mistrust of the hospitals and belief that doctors were little better than "resurrection men" was general.

Rumors also abounded, less traceable to fact, that postmortems had been conducted on the living—that the doctors, in fact, were really burkers themselves, supplying their anatomy subjects from the poor living patient unfortunate enough to end up in the hospital.[11] Finally, the practice of hasty burial of cholera victims, often carried out in a manner considered disrespectful, struck hard at deep cultural investments in funerary practices, including watching and waking, which required that the dead be allowed to lie in the home for several days[12]—although tact on the part of local governments could defuse some potentially difficult situations. Physician Thomas Shapter, in his memoir of the epidemic, relates that, in Exeter in 1832, a difficulty arose when the Jewish community objected to their members being buried in the (Anglican) cholera burial ground. Unprepared for this exigency, and uncertain what their obligations were, the Board of Health managed to be strategically unaware of the one Jewish cholera death, and that victim was duly buried in the Jewish cemetery (170).

The town's tribute to the medical profession in Exeter after the epidemic of 1832 was perhaps partially spurred by a desire to make reparation for the hostility of the poor toward doctors. Shapter's memoir documents not only riots attending hasty removal and burial of the poor, but also accusations that the doctors were causing the disease for their own profit, and frequent harassment, threats, and even physical attacks. In addition, riots and protests, both public and in the form of letters, were the normal responses to the proposal of a cholera hospital or burial ground anywhere in the vicinity. Landowners who offered their property for such uses were liable to be threatened or assaulted, and in many cases rescinded their offers. Shapter documents two such cases with letters written to the Board of Health (140, 149). In one case, a grave digger attempting to bury a patient in a newly appointed burial ground was assaulted and his tools broken (Shapter 145).

On some occasions, the grave diggers themselves could hardly be persuaded to handle the caskets (Shapter 173). In the minutes of a meeting of the St. Olave's District Board of Works, it is recorded that "The bodies of those who have died have been removed as speedily as possible, but in the case of the young woman who died in Vine Street, about 200 and [sic] 300 persons collected to prevent the removal of the body. It was, therefore, not persisted in" ("St. Olave's District Board of Works" 4). The *Shoreditch Observer* also cites opposition of people to removal of corpses from private homes to the public mortuary ("The Health of Shoreditch" 3). Of course, doctors were not defenseless. Historian Ruth Richardson tells the story of residents of Paisely who, having found grave-robbing tools near the churchyard, exhumed coffins by force. Finding some empty, and suspecting the doctors of robbing cholera graves for dissection purposes, the crowd rioted, attacking the residences of doctors and the cholera van. Although the only damage was to property, the medical men of the town resigned from all public office, and the poor were refused the use of parish coffins and hearse (Richardson 225–26). One can hardly think of a worse sanitary move during an epidemic, by the standards of the very people involved in making the decisions. Yet the sense of impending class warfare, and the fears for doctors' personal safety it evoked, overrode other concerns. Doctors were feared not only by those who believed in conspiracies, but by those simply apprehensive of contagion. Archibald Robinson, writing in the *Lancet* of his experiences as a doctor aboard the hulks (convict ships) during the epidemic, notes that "The public mind, however, was systematically worked up to this point; so much so, that my own appearance on shore, after four days and four nights incessant labor in the sick wards, was looked on with as much horror as if a mad dog had been in the street" (559).[13]

Another reaction among the lower classes appears, naturally enough, to have been to use humor and defiance in response to the cholera's terrors. Public drunkenness was common enough to rate frequent mention in sermons, memoirs, and histories. Shapter mentions that "the lower orders" believed that brandy had preventive powers, and therefore drunkenness prevailed to an unusual degree. Besides denying the existence of the disease, humor was a way of dealing with the anxiety, and "wanton songs" were sung about cholera (Shapter 201). (Typically, Shapter solemnly tells many tales of those who jeer at the cholera, and then die of it.) In the *City Press*, a staff writer complained,

> Attention is drawn by a correspondent to the fact that at a highly-patronised music-hall in the metropolis the principle [*sic*] subject of a comic speech is the cholera! The dread scourge is, by the facetious person who addresses his buffoonery to the assembled audience, called "Our Cousin, the Cholera, who has paid us a visit to look after the children—little plagues, of whom the poor have too many." Could anything be more revolting than this, even in these times of tolerance of "comic" singers? ("Suggestions for the Prevention" 6)

Humor, satire, and burlesque were also frequent off the stage. In Paris, this included masks for revelers that mimicked the "visage du cholera." Heinrich Heine gave this account of the epidemic in Paris: "Parisians danced with even more gaiety than usual on the boulevards, where one saw masks whose sickly pallor and deformed features mocked the fear of cholera and the disease itself" (quoted in Delaporte 47). In this account, almost certainly apocryphal, one of the revelers removes his mask to reveal the real visage du cholera, and the masqueraders die so fast they are buried in costume (Delaporte 48). In Britain, musical hall performers sang comic songs about the cholera and did dances burlesquing the spasmodic movements of the victims. Shapter writes of the odd contrast between the general silence of the stricken town and the carnival behavior of some inhabitants:

The general silence of the city [Exeter], save when broken by the tolling of the funeral bell . . . was most remarkable; the streets were deserted, the hurried steps of the medical men and their assistants, or of those running to seek their aid, alone were heard, while the one-horse hearse, occasionally passing on its duty, was almost the only carriage to be seen in the usually busy streets. . . . Amid this desolation, the profligacy and drunkenness of the lower orders increased to such an alarming extent, as to become a matter of public remark and censure. Much of this vice was induced, not only by the general excitement prevailing, but by an idea that brandy was a preventative and panacea for the Cholera; and amongst the lower orders nothing was undertaken without previously resorting to it. (241)

Shapter also observes that many (presumably shotgun) weddings were performed after the epidemic (245).

In short, as Durey and others have observed, the poor (to some extent correctly) interpreted the authorities' response to the cholera as a threat to their autonomy. However, as Durey points out, the wide-scale conspiracy theories that dogged the cholera's progress on the continent—theories that involved an entire class or profession (the aristocracy, the doctors) attempting to murder all the poor—did not gain currency in Britain (183–84). In general, the populace was comparatively very law abiding. Few people were injured or killed, compared to France or Russia, and often it was because of a specific perceived injury (e.g., body snatching), rather than the presence of cholera itself. Perhaps this is because reform, against which cholera was often considered to be a diversionary strategy, provided hope of legitimate recourse for the poor and so defused the impetus to revolution. In any case, however, cholera and fears of revolution were linked all over Europe; in France, cholera was called by some conservatives a "revolutionary infection" (Evans, "Epidemics" 135).

CHOLERA AND "THE PEOPLE" AFTER 1832

After 1832, these reactions were far less frequent. However, subsequent to the first epidemic, evidence suggests that the cholera was an event that could be used by the poor and working classes to advantage. Many urbanites took advantage of fear of cholera to report "nuisances" and get action from landlords, as is seen in letters to the Commissioners of Sewers in this period and occasional letters published in the press.[14] Certainly ratepayers accused the poor of taking advantage of the cholera to press various claims, and probably this was at least sometimes the case. In 1866, *The Shoreditch Observer*, as well as other newspapers, notes that the cholera threat was used by some poor people to gain access to water on Sundays. Additionally, the newspaper observes that "Several cases for compensation where clothing, bedding, and &c., had been destroyed by order of the medical officer were dealt with, but one case where it was destroyed by the parties themselves, and without the order of the authorities" could not be addressed ("The Health of Shoreditch" 3). One letter complains of the "disgusting state of Leadenhall market" and begs that it should be inspected "not at a time when it is dressed for inspection." (In his August 28 follow-up to this complaint in the letter books of the Commissioners of Sewers, Inspector John Simon confirmed the condition of the market as a nuisance.) There are other similar letters of complaint, sometimes multiply signed. The Medical Council reports in 1854 that people are concealing illnesses and deaths by cholera: the possibility of offending a landlord, or being liable as a landlord, is mentioned. On the other hand, professionals' need for information could be used as a bargaining chip: "Great difficulty was experienced at several houses [on Broad Street] in obtaining the requisite information. At No. 19, in particular, it could only be extracted on the condition of reporting an alleged neglect by one of the medical gentlemen named by the parish" (General Board of Health, footnote to chart at end of *Appendix*). Finally, doctors complain that medicine disbursed for cholera patients was often stolen, especially brandy.[15]

Of course, for activists and pro-labor organizations and press, cholera was always an occasion for indictment of the irresponsibility of the wealthy. It was perhaps this consistent resistance that, as much as the expense, gave rise to critiques of the house-to-house visitation that became the preferred method for conducting sanitary inspections, not only of housing but of those who dwelt there. Against the invasion of privacy such visitation entailed, sanitarians cited the results, and the probable attitudes of those visited were hotly debated. Dickens's bricklayer in *Bleak House* who "told off" the lady visitor is supposed to represent this hostility, although Dickens's satire is directed more at useless and inappropriate charity than visiting per se. When the officious Mrs. Pardiggle visits, like a "moral policeman," the man of the house, who has "been drunk for three days," makes his famous speech regarding the value of such social work, as he points to the physical conditions in which his family lives: "Look at the water. Smell it! That's wot we drinks. How do you like it and what do you think of gin, instead! . . . [my lodging] is . . . nat'rally dirty, and it's nat'rally onwholesome, and we've had five dirty and onwholesome children, as is all dead infants, and so much the better" (121). He finishes by bragging that he has beaten his wife (122). Letters to the Metropolitan Commissioners of Sewers at mid-century are rife with references of potential hostility to visitors. A letter by a man named Oscar Fox refers to the notion that house visitation would "frighten people into cholera."

On the other hand, the Commissioners of Sewers Committee on Health defended visiting, and denied any hostility from the visited. John Simon, physician and sanitary inspector, in an 1849 letter to the London Committee on Health, writes, the visitors everywhere are met with expressions of the liveliest gratitude. Nothing could be less founded than the impression that the poor would contemplate these domiciliary visits with suspicion and dislike, or view them in any respect as intrusions. Such an impression could only be entertained by persons whose ignorance of the feelings of the poor disposed them to impute to those classes prejudices which essentially belong to a different one. On the contrary, every possible evidence conspires to assure them that the poor of a Christian Country can recognize the voice of Sympathy and Succour, even when it approaches their thresholds without bidding or obligation.

Meteorologist and sanitarian R. D. Grainger, in 1849, defended visitation on more pragmatic grounds: "there is no reason to suppose that the majority [of persons afflicted] ... would have applied for medical relief at all [unless the visitors had been there], as they appeared to be wholly unconscious of the danger they were in; and the visitors discovered the corpses of several persons who had died of cholera without ever having received any medical aid whatever." The emerging emphasis on the habits of the residents as the primary problem, instead of structural nuisances, comes through clearly in these letters. Surveyor to the Commissioners of Sewers William Haywood writes, in a 1849 letter,

> The house visitation both by the police and by your Inspectors is still in operation as actively as ever and I have as much pleasure in stating as proof of its utility that the number of nuisances are daily decreasing[, yet] the necessity for vigourous inspection, however, during the prevalence of disease still exists for although so much has been done yet from the filthy and careless habits of many of the poor inhabitants nuisances generated almost as quickly as it is removed and the many special cases which have been reported to me by the Inspector obliges me to add that in numerous cases the poorer classes appear to be perfectly apathetical as to the effect of their want of individual care and cleanliness and they abuse or neglect the simple and convenient necessaries provided for their use.

By 1866, the cholera was still a lower class disease, and better understanding of its etiology was offset by a belief that the poor were different in kind from the wealthy, susceptible to different diseases and manifesting them differently.[16]

In the responses of radicals, reformers, and the poor, the pervasiveness of the discursive framework set up by pro-establishment churchmen in the first epidemic is evident. In arguing their case, few disregard the terms of cholera's centrality as a sign of national aims, identity, culpability, and so on. Even parody reinforces the original terms of the debate, rather than undercutting them. Although accepting the connection between politics, the social body, nation, and health may have been politically effective at the moment, the diverse groups that would contribute to what we would later call a liberal ideal of government also tacitly accepted a model which would place the body and its health at the center of discourses of nationhood and citizenship. This continued long after the specific religious and political issues that had originally framed it passed from importance and even memory. This emphasis on the body and its care could be both a help and a hindrance to advocates of the working classes. On the one hand, it gave progressive social reformers leverage for educational and medical reforms that were much needed; on the other, it legitimated an unprecedented level of intervention and regulation.

As I have suggested, this discussion, between clergy, sanitarians, and radicals, set the terms of cholera and the diseased or potentially diseased body's centrality to discussions of the nation and the state for considerable time to come. As the first Reform Bill's agitations and anxiety about disestablishment faded, however, the medical profession slowly became central as the interpretive authority on the body, as the clergy renegotiated its position in relation to secular professional authorities. Epidemic disease, and especially cholera, retained an important role in negotiating the public role of the medic. In the next section, I trace some of these developments.

PART II

Medics and Discourses
of Cholera

Men . . . are always surrounded, in air and water, by an atmosphere
of decaying matter, which is given off from their own bodies.
—William Farr, *Vital Statistics*

Life is a holy thing; and if communities throw away the lives of the
individuals who compose them, or make these sickly, short and
miserable, the community will, in some manner, "pay for it."
—Henry Wentworth Acland,
Memoir on the Cholera at Oxford

4

Medics and the Public Sphere

IN PART I, I TRACED HOW MEDICS first moved to supplant the clergy as public interpreters of the social body's ills and to establish the basis of that interpretation on science rather than religion, on the secular rather than the sacred. The line between spiritual and physical health had long been contested by medics and clergy in the cases of individual patients. Yet, it was particularly difficult for medics, long positioned as the ministers of the private, the secular, the intimate, and the individual, to take authority in the realm of the collective and social, which was also public, moral, and political. Whereas the established church in the early nineteenth century had a well-defined role in the structure of the state, which in turn defined the roles of those dissenting churches and radicals who opposed them, medics began the century as an amorphous group of opposing factions with spotty credentialing practices.

Out of this early welter of confusion emerged, by mid-century, an increasingly coherent profession defined by specialization, scientific and surgical models of the body, and a much-improved public image. In order to understand this transformation, and its relation to cholera—a disease that continued to baffle medical expertise until late in the period—it is useful to examine the development of medical understandings of cholera and the body, as well as the emergence of medical professionalism in this period. As medicine consolidated its position as minister to the social body, medics also attempted to reach some consensus on the nature of cholera. A trend toward racializing and gendering the disease, although much contested by contemporaries as scientifically unsupported, evidences the growing tendency of medics in this period to think in racial terms, and to gender racial otherness feminine.

Throughout the mid-nineteenth century, the British medical profession was defining itself as a profession and consolidating its power, especially in terms of public medicine and the sanitary movement. Beginning with the cholera epidemic of 1832, medics found themselves in a position of both unique opportunity and unique responsibility as they struggled for a place in the nascent public health movement. Key to this process was establishing the nature and terms of medical authority in the public sphere, a process that can be clearly traced in medics' struggles with other forms of authority, especially religious. As shown earlier, a brisk and fairly acrimonious dialogue took place in pamphlets, sermons, letters to editors, and so forth as medical and religious "professionals" jockeyed for position and worked out the nuances of what would eventually become a difficult but productive working relationship. This dialogue included attempts to define an appropriate sphere of influence in the lives of patients/parishioners, arguments about the nature and social role of disease, and, more subtly but perhaps most importantly, the nature that governmental organization of knowledge and intervention into individuals' lives would take, as Britain evolved into a modern liberal state. Medics moved into the position of a kind of secular established clergy, taking over the interpretation of the body's health and its relation to God and nation. Medicine became both a public, and later, an elite profession, as its status as an art came to be redefined in terms of science, and Britain came to see itself as a scientific and modern nation. Medical discourses increasingly authorized themselves with the rhetoric of national interest and improvement, and medics used the public attention elicited by cholera to create a public platform for the profession. They mobilized discourses of nation and the social to add force to their position, and in so doing, contributed to the formation of those discourses themselves.

SANITARIANS AND MEDICS

Medics and sanitarians were of course diverse if overlapping groups, and here I would like to unpack at least some of the complexities of the terms. Sanitarians, throughout the century, were often medics who believed in sanitary reform, but also might well be laypersons, such as Edwin Chadwick, with no medical training, for whom sanitary reform seemed a matter of common sense. However, official representation on the Board of Health, and thus public authority for defining the sanitary agenda, does shift over the period from lay authorities such as Chadwick to medics such as physician John Simon and licensed apothecary William Farr. The term "medics" comprises four ill-defined groups at the beginning of the century. The first three were the traditional ones: physicians, graduates of universities, and usually gentlemen who dealt with physic, that is, illnesses of the interior of the body that were thought to require an understanding of its systems; surgeons, who dealt with the exterior of the body, wounds, and so forth; and apothecaries, who dispensed drugs and early on, frequently prescribed them and attended patients either with minor illnesses or those who could not afford physicians. Physicians, early in the period, held a view of physic in which illness was seen as an imbalance of systems involving the whole body. Surgeons and apothecaries, especially the latter, were sometimes considered tradesmen at this time. Surgeons were supposed to deal with what were considered "local affections," illnesses or injuries localized in a particular part of the body, not requiring the intervention or expertise of the physician. Apothecaries dispensed drugs and advice and often also duplicated the more minor work of surgeons—small surgeries, bonesetting, and so forth—among the poor.

These professional distinctions were classed (one thinks of Jane Eyre, who, with the servants, is treated by the local apothecary whereas the children of the mistress are treated by a physician). Neither surgeons nor apothecaries, at the end of the eighteenth century, would have had a diploma. They relied instead on an apprenticeship system and sometimes also attended private lectures. But medical "reform" was already a topic of debate long before the advent of the cholera, and encompassed both the need for more stringent licensing practices and the need for structural change in the profession reflecting new scientific information. After 1800, surgeons in England were able to take an exam providing certification, and after 1815, apothecaries were licensed through the Society of Apothecaries. By the early 1830s, the rising importance of anatomical medicine and its prevalence in Paris meant that many aspiring surgeons who had the means would attend lectures there; the subject matter subsequently became popular in London. In 1836, the University of London started to confer medical degrees and constituted a Board of Examiners that could confer licenses to surgeons; subsequently, other colleges also began to offer courses in surgical medicine. Therefore, by the mid-century, surgeons were more likely to study at specifically medical schools than were physicians, attending lectures and anatomy classes, as well as serving apprenticeships in hospitals. Still, standardization and policing of such practices did not become widespread until considerably later. Predictably, the distinctions between kinds of practitioner were clearer in theory than in practice, and probably for many patients in the middling-to-lower classes, they were largely meaningless. Even after these licenses were available to surgeons and apothecaries, many practitioners did not undergo licensure or the training it required. They simply hung out their shingles when they felt adequately trained, though they were not entitled to use the letters FRCS (Fellow of the Royal College of Surgeons) or LSA (Licentiate of the Society of Apothecaries) after their names. In the fourth category, there were also various midwives, nurses, and other female practitioners, and a range of "quacks" who, though formally untrained, were often trusted medical advisors with much practical experience, as well as those who simply defrauded the public, knowingly selling useless potions and pills.

Complicating these distinctions further was the changing status of surgical medicine as medical theories and technologies changed (and also the fact that many practitioners in the vast middling ranks of the profession combined treatment styles). Historian Christopher Lawrence has demonstrated the connection between the increased value of anatomical knowledge and the rising status of the surgeon in the mid-century, whose techniques were increasingly invasive of the body's interior, even before anesthesia (24).[1] Surgeons were positioned, argues Lawrence, as manly, heroic, "democratic heroes," as opposed to an effete notion of physic. In any case, even as early as the 1830s, surgeons were violating the boundaries of their supposed domain—the body's exterior and extremities—and certainly used (and even dispensed) drugs also, which were supposedly the domain of the apothecary. The surgical tendency toward specialization, as opposed to the physician's broader systemic view of the body, provided a means of legitimation and market competition by mid-century, as well as establishing exclusion of other practitioners.[2] Physicians, meanwhile, by the late 1840s were increasingly likely to be interested in surgical models of medicine, though they tended to continue to subordinate those models to physic.

Early on, the combination of treatment methods was reflected by the number of medics identifying as surgeon-apothecaries, who dispensed drugs, advised, dressed wounds, performed surgery, and cared for fevers all at once.[3] It was only wealthy families who could afford both a physician and a surgeon in attendance. The surgeon-apothecaries, licensed both by the LSA and the FRCS, were a manifestation of what would come to be known as general practitioners, a non-official designation that emerged in the early part of the century (which later became an official descriptor). As historian Irvine Loudon demonstrates, although the surgeon per se rose in status, the general practitioner became the lower-grade medic most people consulted for ordinary health problems. This was especially the case after the '50s, as specialization became increasingly important to professional identity.

Specialization became a way of legitimating authority through knowledge instead of social background, as Jeanne Peterson has demonstrated. Specialization was largely the tool of the surgeon (though occasionally, general practitioners would declare a "specialized" practice). Thus, it was a powerful tool for upward mobility. Physicians at first loathed and resisted the surgical specialists, whose work was a serious economic threat, and moreover, was incompatible with the systemic view of physic upon which physicians' identity rested. As late as the 1860s, physicians launched a serious attack on surgical specialists (Peterson 273–74). Still, by that time, these surgeons were thoroughly established and popular with the public (Peterson 264). Specialists used specialty hospitals, organizations, and perhaps most importantly, journals, to consolidate their power and status through shared knowledge and networking. In the first forty years of the nineteenth century, almost three times the number of new journals were launched than in the 160 years preceding (Bartrip 8). In short, all the groups of medics, but especially the three "below" the physicians, display an increasing professionalization, defined by internal regulation, closure (limitation of access to professional status), and self-legitimation based on exclusive and shared knowledge. By the '60s, physicians had largely come to accept and integrate an understanding of the body that included "special pathology," or the study of individual diseases and bodily ailments, and recognized the importance of anatomical study—a testimony to the power of the surgical approach.

SANITARIANS UNDER CHADWICK

The early lay sanitarians, under Edwin Chadwick, were dismissive of or even hostile to expert medical opinion. The sanitary movement, which focused on the notion that disease was caused by filth and directed its energies to cleaning up "nuisances," like foul drains, dunghills, and the like, began as a movement of laypersons. Chadwick had no medical training and initially did not see the necessity of including medics in the movement. He subsequently did include medics: physicians Thomas Southwood Smith, James Kay-Shuttleworth, and Neil Arnott. As Margaret Pelling notes, Chadwick's three medics became, through institutional control of information dissemination, the "official" voices on the cholera early on—this created a false impression of anti-contagionism, both for the public and for historians later (7). The reality was more complex, as has been ably documented by many scholars since Margaret Pelling's path-breaking study. First, Chadwick's doctors were dismissive of the state of medical knowledge in the profession, especially the contrarian Southwood Smith. Sanitarians were broadly anti-contagionist, but that was by no means the mainstream medical opinion—in fact, the profession was probably about evenly split on the matter. There were also, especially by mid-century, a whole range of compromise positions along a spectrum from contagionism to anti-contagionism. But as the *Lancet*, which was, under Wakley, contagionist on the cholera issue, bitterly remarked of those who held this view, "Every man who dared to speak the truth was pointed out as the enemy of this country and its commerce" (Editors 571).

As historian Christopher Hamlin has very eloquently shown, Chadwick was highly motivated to find that filth, rather than either contagion or deprivation, was the primary cause of disease among the poor. Because he was the architect of the New Poor Law, suspicions that the poor were starved or malnourished, and that this scarcity was what made them so vulnerable to disease, seemed an indictment of his system. (The system that Chadwick had devised provided that any truly destitute person could apply for relief through admittance to the poor house—hence, no one need starve. But in so doing, the person gave up freedom and any remnant of respectability, and had to endure what were widely felt to be harsh conditions, and so the poor houses were often avoided by the people they were intended to serve.) Chadwick was often at odds with local medical officers who stubbornly listed "want" as a proximate cause of death (Hamlin, *Public Health*). Further, although parish doctors had to supply drugs at their own expense, the parish paid for food—hence it was cheaper for medical officers to medicate with food than drugs (Hamlin, *Public Health* 95; see also Digby 246–47). Chadwick wanted workhouses to be perceived by the poor as worse than the generally inadequate living conditions outside; at the same time, he had to present them to the public as a rational and humane solution to pauperism. This dual aim required a kind of constant brinksmanship between Malthusianism and Benthamism, between starvation of the inmates and a too-humane care (Hamlin, *Public Health* 33). Thus, although Chadwick's three physicians, all ideologically committed to the belief that poverty was avoidable through individual effort, found filth to be *the* public health problem in Britain, radical *Lancet* editor Thomas Wakley and Chartist leader William Lovett found hunger to be the chief evil (Hamlin, *Public Health* 86). As Hamlin notes, many medics were critical of Chadwick's point of view, seeing poverty and want as systemic evils, productive of disease themselves. Political radicals and their sympathizers systematically took this critical view, as seen in the "Feast Day" response to the public fast occasioned by the first cholera epidemic. Chadwick went so far as to claim that an austere diet was healthier than a richer one (Hamlin, *Public Health* 96). Still, to Chadwick's dismay, even Kay-Shuttleworth refused to denounce the parish medical men who prescribed food, out of professional courtesy (Hamlin, *Public Health* 95).

Chadwick's moralizing attitude toward poverty implied a set of values that defined the question of poverty as a social one and therefore explicitly not economic or political in nature. Of Chadwick's three medical men, James Kay-Shuttleworth has garnered, perhaps, the most attention. His tract emerging from his work in the 1832 epidemic in Manchester, *The Moral and Physical Condition of the Working Classes Employed in the Cotton Manufacture in Manchester*, was foundational for the Manchester Statistical Society. As John Pickstone and Mary Poovey have both pointed out, this tract is a good example of the articulation of the social body metaphor. The entire text is framed in body imagery. Kay-Shuttleworth proposes the construction of an artificial "afferent nervous system"—that is, statistical medical monitoring—to convey to the "thinking" portion of the population the condition of the animalized poor, who suffer without intellectual understanding or the ability to communicate.[4] Urban Britain, he charges, is a degenerate organism: "The sensorium of the animal structure . . . is endowed with a consciousness of every change in the sensations to which each member is liable. . . . Pain thus reveals to us the existence of evils, which, unless arrested in their progress, might insidiously invade the sources of vital action" (17), but unfortunately society's body lacks that "pervading consciousness" (18). Historian John Pickstone observes of this text that

> The theorizing of the poor as a separate mass was conditioned not only by their acquiring a separate voice, but by their increasingly separate geographic existence . . . hence the power of Kay's medical imagery where he compared the working-class area to regions of the body; regions which may be diseased without the cognisance of the higher centres. . . . In that image there is not only distance, but lack of mutuality. (411)

Because communication is slow or lacking over this distance, statistical investigations were needed to act as the "afferent nervous system through which the social body could feel pain. The degeneration of this nerveless part of the social body was at once a moral, political and medical threat" (Pickstone 411).

As Mary Poovey notes, the authority of Kay-Shuttleworth's representation of the poor originates in the language of anatomy and dissection. He uses this authority to position cholera and indeed poverty as subject to amelioration by middle-class social intervention, rather than political activism (Poovey 60). As Poovey has also noted, Kay-Shuttleworth uses the social body as a representation of nation, in order to deflect critique of capitalism and its ills. He places blame instead on the Irish (about whom Kay-Shuttleworth is unusually virulent), and expresses anxiety about the inappropriate domesticity of working-class women. Characteristically, these domestic inadequacies lead to a vague "licentiousness" (Kay-Shuttleworth 62) and the decline of religion, which is the ineffable soul of the social body: "The absence of religious feeling . . . ensure[s] a concomitant civic debasement. The social body cannot be constructed like a machine, on abstract principles which merely include physical motions. . . . Political economy . . . cannot accomplish its design, without . . . the cultivation of religion and morality" (Kay-Shuttleworth 63–64).

Kay-Shuttleworth's tract starts off sounding much like Marx (or Adam Smith, for that matter):

> prolonged and exhausting labour . . . is not calculated to develop the intellectual or moral faculties of man. The dull routine of a ceaseless drudgery, in which the same mechanical process is incessantly repeated, resembles the torment of Sisyphus. . . . The intellect slumbers . . . but the grosser parts of our nature attain a rank development. To condemn man to such severity of toil is . . . to cultivate in him the habits of an animal. (20–22)

He comes to the conclusion that such a worker "lives in squalid recklessness, on meager food and expends his superfluous gains in debauchery" (22). Kay-Shuttleworth accuses this Irish worker of setting an example which, strangely, the English worker finds so compelling that he follows the Irishman's lead: that is, he accepts a mere subsistence level of wages and spends it on drink when he has a bit more. All this leads to the worker's neglect of domesticity, and from there, Kay-Shuttleworth arrives at the deracination of the English. Fortunately for the cotton magnates of Manchester, Kay-Shuttleworth assures them, capitalism is not the cause. In fact, capitalism is itself threatened by this Irish illness: "The evils affecting the working classes, *so far from being the necessary results of the commercial system, furnish evidence of a disease which impairs its energies, if it does not threaten its vitality*" (Kay-Shuttleworth's emphasis, 79).

From this point on in the essay, Kay-Shuttleworth's position is that of the typical mid-century middle-class liberal—educate the people specially in domestic economy, and an "enlightened popular opinion" (96), illuminated by "*cheap treatises*" with "*correct* political information" (his emphasis, 96–97), would eventually incorporate them into what we would call a middle-class public sphere. As Poovey puts it, Kay-Shuttleworth equates "national well-being with the economic health of a newly politicized, respectable middle class" (72).[5] Chadwick, although not so motivated to marginalize the Irish, essentially fostered the same split between economic and social reality: capitalism did not cause poverty or hunger, and anyway, hunger wasn't such a bad thing. Poovey observes that what really mattered for Chadwick was to have women who were appropriately domestic, and for men to define themselves through that domesticity rather than through homosocial relationships which might lead to political action. This ensured "that a man's most significant same-sex relationship would be formed through his wife to himself—to his 'character'" (her emphasis, 125). These constructions of domesticity and labor were inextricable from discussions of the Poor Law and debates on workers' fitness for the franchise. In short, from the beginning, sanitary choices were inseparable from political positions on reform and the Poor Law.

Chadwick was quick enough to discount even his own employees' medical advice as politically beside the point when it came to actual social engineering. When Yorkshire physician Charles Loudon had stated that no one should work more than ten hours per day in a factory, Chadwick, whose concern was only the limitation of hours for children, noted that Loudon was speaking "merely 'as a physician.'" Of course, he stated, such concerns could not override "moral and social considerations which discountenance all legislative interference with the disposal of labour extending beyond the age of childhood" (quoted in Hamlin, *Public Health* 99). He also attacked medical credibility based on personal experience with cases by referring to statistical models that would require data from multiple locations and practitioners

(Hamlin, *Public Health* 100). For Chadwick's men, medicine and politics were to be separable at need into airtight containers, and indeed, his coworker, Neil Arnott, attacked positions he disagreed with by arguing that their science was corrupt because politicized (Hamlin, *Public Health* 143).[6] Yet, Chadwick's work was quite overtly political. Chadwick positioned himself against Chartism and democracy in favor of sanitation as a project of social control (Hamlin, *Public Health* 185–86). As Hamlin shows, Chadwickian pragmatism aligned public health much more with broad sanitary and housing reform—largely affairs of urban management, rather than medicine.

So although there were medics involved in Chadwick's regime, in part to legitimate it to the medical profession (a concession that already showed considerable gain for medics), the ones he chose were by no means necessarily representative of the larger profession's views. In fact, the medics working with Chadwick were frequently politically positioned against many of their colleagues. Still, many medics did agree early on with the sanitary idea, and some used it and the cholera epidemics, as well as the structure of Poor Law medicine, to launch their own careers in public administration, such as Thomas Shapter of Exeter. Many of even the *Lancet*'s readers identified as did one correspondent, "although I am Tory to the backbone in General Politics, I am radical to the heart's core in Medical Politics" (quoted in Loudon 131)—a position with many logical contradictions, but not untenable in a well-compartmentalized social life. Such political positioning generally, though not by any means always, correlated with class. It was the rising groundswell of middle- and lower-middle-class practitioners, often surgeon-apothecaries, who forced the issue of medical reform and professionalization. Often they began their careers with politically radical or at least liberal beliefs, but as aspirants to the upper levels of the bourgeoisie, they, too, had reasons to espouse more conservative values.

THE PROFESSION OF MEDICINE: FROM PRIVATE TO PUBLIC

The emergence of professionalism was defined in part by closure and exclusion. Admittance to the profession required agreement about the nature of the profession—a definition of a shared and specialized body of knowledge to be applied in a standard way (a shared "product"). This called for a shared educational process and some mechanism of certification. Usually, professional organizations descended from the ancient guilds that represented the interests of the group and also arbitrated disputes having to do with professional definition.[7] Marxist theorists such as Magali Larson have emphasized the way in which knowledge was made exclusive in order to create a power base and economic monopoly. This historically specific project has generally been founded on the truth claims of science, and often appeals to the state for legitimation. In medicine's case, this was achieved in part by positioning the profession as integral to state power. As Roy Lewis and Angus Maude note, the project of professionalizing medicine involved the establishment of codes of conduct and ethics with some claim of broader public service (56). As they also point out, however, the inviolability of the personal client-practitioner relationship often conflicts with a broader notion of public service, as does the sense that the professional's first responsibility is to the client who has paid for one's services (59–64): "So important is the practitioner-client relationship to the historical and conventional conception of professional ethics, that it is sometimes suggested that only private practice confers professional status" (61).

Yet, of course, in their links to the state, the professions have indeed been involved in public affairs from at least the mid-nineteenth century, and in some cases, (law and the clergy, for example), much earlier. Medicine is interesting, however, for its development in both directions at once and its meteoric shift from a profession very much in the private sphere at the beginning of the century to one with considerable public responsibility by the '60s. Peterson has noted that, unlike the other professions, fewer than twenty percent of medical men came from the upper classes; it was in many ways seen as a subservient profession and medics had to fight hard to establish social status. As professionals financially dependent upon clients, Victorian general practitioners, at least, tended to network by joining sports and music clubs, but eschewed politics, "some even to the point of refusing to vote" (Peterson 128). Since authority in the early to mid century, according to Peterson, came not from medical knowledge but from "connections, social origin, or social style," few lower-middle-class general practitioners could afford to jeopardize it by deviating from the expected norm (134). Both Harriet Martineau, in her novel *Deerbrook*, and George Eliot, in *Middlemarch*, dramatize the ethical and social difficulties associated with this conflict between dependency and public obligation; in both novels, medical men's professional lives collide with their political and social connections, injuring them economically and socially.

James Eli Adams has suggested that the connection between gender and class identity was destabilized by the new class mobility in the early nineteenth century. Of course this especially affected the medical profession, whose class investments were changing so rapidly. Professions dealing largely in the private sphere could be seen as gender ambiguous or feminized, as their class attachments were called into question. Medicine, involving the intimate care of the body, was a profession deeply entrenched in the most private areas of life. This was one reason that the highest rank of the profession, physicians, often only consulted verbally without touching the body, never administering medicine themselves, in the early years of the century. Theoretical knowledge of the body was a matter for a gentleman, but physical manipulation of the body was too much like manual work—or nursing. Moving into the public sphere, through the mediating structure of the social domain, enabled surgeons and general practitioners to establish their masculinity. Indeed, the 1858 Act, which standardized the profession and drew the four major groups under one rubric, eliminated women from the profession entirely, severely limiting what midwives could do and definitively excluding women from certification by establishing conditions impossible for women to meet institutionally in Britain. In scholars' focus on the Dr. Lydgates of history, it can be forgotten that Felix Holt and even Sairy Gamp were medics as well, who often delivered much the same services as physicians and surgeons, despite differences in class and social status, until 1858.[8] The very concept of womanhood as belonging to the private and private-social spheres disallowed the concept of publicity associated with late nineteenth-century professionalism.[9]

Regardless of the struggles over hierarchical stratification within ranks, medicine was, as a whole, presenting an increasingly coherent and professional face to the world and basing its claims upon an ideal of social centrality and service to the *nation*, defined not simply as interests of the state or of an elite but as the interests of an inclusive social body whose claims upon the state-as-nation were perceived as both standing separate from and exceeding political and class interests. Specialization and professionalism encouraged medics who lacked the connections, wealth, and background to be traditional physicians to draw on their strengths and apply them to public health and epidemic medicine. Parish appointments and medical officer berths enabled young medics (especially surgeons) of middle- and lower-middle-class background to gain training and prove themselves as public servants, entering a different level of social status and gaining a voice in community affairs.

The emergence of medicine as a "public" profession was thus complex and depended much on a clear definition of what one means by "public." One example from Christopher Hamlin's excellent study of public health may serve to illustrate. Hamlin notes that as early as 1823, a medic writing in Burnett's *Medical Advisor* expressed outrage at the treatment of a nursing mother who was put to the treadmill in prison and took it for granted that it was specifically medical authority that gave him the right of judgment (*Public Health* 17). Hamlin also mentions that "doctors," by speaking to their friends who were powerful officials and would have seen the controversy in the newspapers, would quickly put an end to such abuses. Hamlin argues that this shows the clear sense that medics were appropriately engaged in questions of public politics and expected to be active (*Public Health* 17). However, I would use the same episode to point out that medics were positioned very much as a middle-class woman might be; outraged by a question of cruelty, they wrote on the subject, mobilized public feeling, and influenced powerful men to act. They did not yet, however, ask for a medical officer to be consulted every time a policy issue was at stake. It was still a "social" rather than a political question.

The "social" was the domain that mediated between the public and private in order to create and sustain that fictional division. Various theorists have placed the onset of the social as a separate category at times ranging from the late 1700s to the early 1900s.[10] However, the period in which it becomes possible to define the social both as a field and a problem is in the nineteenth century. The social was perhaps most decisively inaugurated as a public and legislative issue in 1834, with the passage of the New Poor Law.[11] Society, in popular parlance, designated the arena of relations between and within (elite) families: friendship, courtship, and all the alliances on which business and community were based. The more specific use of the term "social," as it was elaborated in this period, was what Victorians used to define "social problems" and we have come to associate with "social work": interventions into the lives of the poor, especially conceived as poor *families*, in order to correct problems largely conceived of as inadequate socialization. The two uses were thus not unrelated; social work sought to produce the values believed to be basic to society in a class that was seen as having insufficiently developed them.

Mary Poovey, who has given the most provocative elucidation of the social body in the early Victorian period, places the development of the social in the late 1700s, allying it with the development of statistical and theoretical representations of populations as aggregates. This time period, according to Poovey, corresponded with the first clear sense of the social sphere as distinct from the domains of economics and politics:

> These two developments—the aggregation of distinct populations and the conceptual disaggregation of a social domain—were intimately connected, for identifying the problems that afflicted the nation involved isolating the offending populations, abstracting from individual cases the general problems they shared, and devising solutions that would not contradict the specific rationalities of those domains by which British social relations had traditionally been organized. (8)

At the same time, Poovey notes, it was fundamental to "political rationality" that political power should be based in the ownership of property, even as it was increasingly widely believed that trade and commerce should be liberated from governmental interference (8). Therefore, the appearance of the social as a separate domain was associated with "the specification of a set of problems that was related to but not coincident with political and economic issues" (Poovey 8). The social was also associated with femininity: the intimacy of bodily processes and domesticity. By redefining problems of poverty, poor hygiene, and disease as social problems rather than economic ones, these problems became susceptible to social solutions focusing on the education of poor women who were perceived as primarily responsible for the home environments of their husbands and children. To this end, social work became an extension of philanthropic activities in which women took a large role: home visiting, for example. They worked in tandem with medics and clergy.

Hamlin argues that, because medical matters "were matters of political and social relations, they were inescapably public." However, since the "social" was constituted as a vexed area between public and private, and at base, under the direct ministration of a feminine and feminized intervention, it was not, at this time, in the public sphere. Susan Lawrence has argued that eighteenth-century hospital teaching and the publication of early journals constituted a public professional presence (23), and to some extent this was so, in the sense that within the profession there was a limited public within which knowledge was constituted, and that journals helped pave the way for medics to have a wider sense of presence and community (see esp. 271–76). However, this is not "public" in the sense that I use it here: that is, in the Habermasian sense of a public sphere having to do with constitution of a critical citizenry responding to functions of state. As Lawrence acknowledges, medics of the eighteenth century saw their knowledge as apolitical and quite distinct from "public matters" per se. Only later did social (or medical) issues become public ones, and that took place with the advancement of official, professional positions having to do with its oversight. The public health movement is part of this history of the governmentalization of social issues.[12]

The "pre-Chadwickian paradigm" of public health that Hamlin finds from 1790–1840 (*Public Health* 23) was a fascinating and important part of the groundwork that aligned health with the social and prepared the way for a redefinition of the social as a "quasi-public" domain of knowledge and intervention. As Hamlin himself later notes, medical men only advised, never mandated; unlike the other great medieval professions, medicine was not public, "to practice medicine was not to make health policy: medicine was a private profession," and its "focus . . . was the person, not policy, and balance, not . . . change" (*Public Health* 50). But he is certainly right that the "great social issues" were "significantly medical" (*Public Health* 25). In this period, the secular professions' ideal of "public" service was predominantly in the realm of the "social," and the social itself was not yet fully public in the sense we commonly use the term. The concept of a social body identical with a nation which was also a population, rather than a set of political or "state" interests, became in this century more or less coterminous with the "social" domain in which these professionals exercised their authority. This created an odd division. In the performance of their professional duties, they were seen as belonging to the realm of the social, and therefore apolitical. But as the social became more central to the aims of government, social experts became newly important. To the extent that these professionals published (or spoke publicly) on matters of policy, informed by their social expertise, they were public figures, even though what they spoke about were seen essentially as private matters. Inevitably, such matters were caught up in political questions, as the scope of tax-supported "charity" widened.

CHADWICK'S SUCCESSORS: JOHN SIMON AND WILLIAM FARR

The rise of John Simon and William Farr did much more than Chadwick had done to align medical and sanitary interests at the administrative level. Simon was trained as a surgeon, and Farr had continental training that was basically surgical in nature, though he was licensed only as an apothecary. Simon, who succeeded Chadwick and was appointed the first Chief Medical Officer for England in 1855, managed to "eliminate the gap between that [sanitary] doctrine and the profession as a whole" (Pelling 230). He stood upon the need for a professional medic to determine sanitary policy—a welcome move to most medics after the brusquerie of Chadwick. Farr's role in the Office of the Registrar-General was even more crucial to the epistemological shift in public health in favor of medicalization and statistic modeling. In 1836, the Registrar-General's office was created in order to keep track of statistical matters, including medical information such as mortality rates. Farr became the "compiler of abstracts," a position that he was to hold for the next forty-two years. Hamlin observes that Farr challenged Chadwick by aligning himself with those who saw starvation as a sanitary problem (*Public Health* 145).[13]

The first three cholera epidemics had been publicly handled within the rubric of the sanitary movement. Regardless of the internecine wars about contagionism, appropriate treatment, the seat of the disease, among other things, *publicly* and in terms of policy the disease was a filth disease, a sanitary disease, not contagious but infectious. Soon after the third epidemic, the power of both Simon as the leader of the official sanitary bureaucracy and Farr in the Registrar-General's office promoted a closer and more decisive identification between the medical profession and sanitation. By the fourth epidemic, new coherence in medical theories, and perhaps, the success of the sanitary project in meeting many of its goals, allowed even public discussion of the disease largely to become medicalized. Medics accepted the importance of sanitation in controling disease; however, disease was also discussed in terms of its hidden etiology and dependence upon human actions. Some of this was as a result of international pressure after the International Cholera Conference of 1866 decided that the blame for worldwide pandemics should be laid on the British authorities who governed Bengal, which had been identified as the source of the disease.[14] However, it was also as a result of gains in professional influence—the sanitary movement was being managed more by medics than previously. In part because experts like Simon and Farr provided the bridge by which medics were brought into sanitary management as a regular part of their duties, through mortality returns and the like, medics were enabled to make the leap from interpreters of individual bodies to groups, which allowed them to claim a stake in public management and politics.

Farr represents an unusual class background. A working-class orphan, he came under the patronage of a master who provided him with education. Historian Margaret Pelling states that Farr "was [not] ever part of the medical profession" (111); that is true in terms of individual practice, but certainly not in the broader sense of training and participation in the public shaping of the profession. He had a typical general practitioner's background: he "studied medicine with a physician, served as dresser to a surgeon, and was 'nominally apprenticed' to an apothecary" (Eyler 1). He also studied morbid anatomy in Paris, where he was exposed to the study of hygiene and medical statistics (Eyler 2). (In Paris, medicine had professionalized much earlier—although stratified, it was publicly regulated and already a recognized part of the state apparatus by the early 1800s.) Although better trained than most physicians of his time by today's standards, Farr returned to Britain licensed only as an apothecary, and turned to medical journalism to make a living (Eyler 2–3). Farr's early writings showed a preoccupation with the professional and social aspects of medicine: as he wrote in 1839, "Profession is here understood to imply the history of a social institution, established to preserve the health and alleviate the physical sufferings of the nation" (in Eyler 3). Farr, a close associate of *Lancet* editor Thomas Wakley, believed in medical reform and democratization; he also believed, as aforementioned, in the profession as an institution that had a public role to play in the regulation of national affairs. He had a thorough trust in science and an environmental approach to public health congenial with that of the sanitarians. He also conceived public health in terms of race, eugenics, and degeneration, which was to provide an important platform for public health after the first wave of the sanitary movement.

Farr's forty-two years of work as a statistician for the Registrar-General's office began in 1839, and he crafted that position into a powerful site from which to create and disseminate knowledges of public health. With far less investment in the Poor Law than Chadwick, Farr was well positioned to denounce the lack of medical care and basic necessaries of life the poor suffered, and he did. Yet, he too found pauperism morally objectionable and believed in moral environmentalism—in his eyes, pauperism created moral as well as physical evil.[15] Good sanitarian *and* good medic, Farr created a context and discourse within which medics—especially general practitioners—could more comfortably work within the sanitary movement and claim it as their own. For the general public, there was already little doubt by this time that the medical point of view was also the sanitary point of view.

Farr's other great contribution was to firmly root the connection between the already lively medical interest in statistics with a formal institutional position and a public health agenda. Statistics enabled medics to leap from diagnosis of the individual patient to the larger questions of populations that justified their speaking in the public interest. The sanitary movement (and the advent of widespread vaccination) enabled them to *prescribe* for populations, and this was an important point. It was not enough merely to be able to observe that certain districts were healthy or unhealthy, or even to say that something specific in a district caused disease—medics had been doing that kind of medical topography for years, but such observations could only lead to individual diagnoses. A single sick patient could be advised to leave an unhealthy area, but entire populations could not practically be so treated. The sanitary movement, however, allowed medics to prescribe for populations—for a *public*—by tackling the question of how to treat "sick" environments. Farr's creation of the classification of "zymotic" diseases, the presence of which acted as an index of public morbidity, designated a type of disease by its appropriateness for intervention that was both specifically medical and specifically public.[16] Zymotic disease collapsed previously discreet categories such as epidemic, endemic, and contagious disease, linking all as having to do with putrifying matter.

On the other hand, Farr's nosology also facilitated the surgical desire for "specific pathologies"—that is, for the location of disease in a particular site.[17] Additionally, whereas Chadwick argued that anyone with a working olfactory sense could detect sites for sanitary interventions, Farr based his determinations on medical theory not available to the layman, even while retaining the basic sanitary framework of filth-generation. Farr also provided a bridge between the camps of contagionism and anti-contagionism (positions that maintained that the cholera either was or was not spread through human contact, of which more later). In short, Farr subscribed to a modified version of the contingent contagionism, which had become the dominant via media for many professionals, disregarding the hard-line sanitarian anti-contagionism of Southwood-Smith and Chadwick that had created needless antagonism with most medics who could not agree with it.[18]

Farr's work with population density, altitude, and ventilation was important to housing reformers who were concerned with separating bodies believed to give off what he called "zymotic" material with every respiration— roughly, material that, like fermenting substances, could reproduce itself by transforming surrounding matter. For Farr, even healthy bodies were vectors of illness: as I discuss in chapter 5, this belief placed his views in line with the emergence of new medical theories influenced by French developments in pathology. Early on, Farr linked these questions to issues of racial degeneration, which he believed was a national threat. The concentration of bodies giving off zymotic materials could cause entire populations, and their offspring, to decline. Not only did these developments enable the sanitary movement to continue a lively business in housing reform beyond the duration of projects of sewerage and street cleaning, but, again, they shifted the questions of sanitation to the grounds of expert medical and engineering knowledge, professionalizing them. In an 1866 letter to the *City Press*, Robert Fowler, M.D., District Medical Officer of the East London Union, justifies raising wages for medical officers by arguing that "The very great importance to the Public Health of the information that the Poor Law Medical Officers are alone capable of affording may be amply illustrated by any member of the Court of Sewers. . . . I venture to assert that the Commissioners of Sewers have never heretofore received such reports. They contain data and facts such as would be collated by skilled observers alone" (3). By the end of his life, even though he had always been suspicious of authoritarian institutional solutions, Farr came to recommend quite stringent government intervention in biomanagement. Farr, of course, was not the only or even the most influential of the sanitary reformers of the mid-century. But his work represents a significant shift that enabled a smooth merging of the medical and sanitary projects into one larger public health endeavor, made possible in part by the idea of professionalization as bearing social meanings and responsibilities as well as relying on specialized knowledge.

MEDICS PRESCRIBING MORALITY

Finally, despite medics' struggle to claim a specifically medical ground from which to speak on public affairs, Victorians' firm conviction that physical and moral hygiene were intertwined contributed to both medics' and clergy's claims to speak about health issues—with due respect for each other's differing areas of expertise.

Moral health and physical health cannot be separated in this era: in the '30s it was thought that cholera struck populations that were immoral and excessive in their habits, and by the '50s it was still largely believed that insanitary environments resulted as much, if not more, from the habits of those who lived within them as of infrastructure or economics. One of the ironies of the period is that as public health was secularized, and clergy became the handmaidens of the new science, medics' public position enabled them to hold forth on wider questions of morality as being scientifically and medically based. For example, in his *Memoir on the Cholera at Oxford in the Year 1854*, published in 1856, physician and Oxford professor of medicine Henry Wentworth Acland uses the medical bully pulpit to make a number of broader points, claiming a social authority that extends to the moral domain. Part 3 of his *Memoir*, "The Lesson of the Epidemic," begins with a rhetoric not dissimilar from that of sermons on the national fast days for the first two cholera epidemics, which emphasized the relation between individual responsibility and national sin, though with a sanitary twist:

> Instances of individual self-destruction from avoidable circumstances might be multiplied without end. With these individual cases we have not here to deal. Each man has a free will, and he must make his choice according to the knowledge he possesses. But with communities this is not so: they have lawgivers and laws . . . it is not to be doubted . . . that [civilized] *communities*, as well as *individuals*, may violate the sanitary laws which our Creator has imposed on us; and that the consequence of the violation of these laws is punishment to the *community* for its *common* crime; as it is in the case of the individual for his individual crime. . . . Life is a holy thing; and if communities throw away the lives of the individuals who compose them, or make these sickly, short and miserable, the community will, in some manner, "pay for it." (Acland's emphases, 105–06)

There follows a Utilitarian argument about paying rates to support the disabled and orphaned.

Although he carefully separates the individual and the community, it seems quite clear from elsewhere in his argument, as he exhorts the sanitary authorities to use their powers to force remediation, that the individual's right to exercise that free will should be severely limited when it impacts the larger community. In turn, the community is represented, not by a composite of individual wills, but by the more powerful wills of its lawgivers and rulers. His argument evokes the rhetoric of natural laws and general providence, though he stays within the utilitarian rather than the moral rhetoric much of the time. Indeed, it should not be surprising to find language similar to sermons on national sin and disease as punishment, published in response to the first epidemic, here. Medics (and other sanitarians) often used public discourse in the same way that clergy used sermons, to define a community that was inclusive of all classes and that showed the interdependence of the well-to-do reader with the lower classes most likely to suffer from the disease—or be part of the conditions to spread it. In his summary of the book's argument, he defends the inclusion of the lengthy third section and also its limits in language that evokes England's vision of itself as "civilized" with mild irony:

> To enumerate the arrangements which a wise Community would adopt beforehand to mitigate the terrible scourge of coming Epidemics, would be

to describe the manner in which a civilized and well-regulated people, acquainted with the laws of health and the causes of disease, would strive to live on ordinary occasions: and as this would lead the reader into questions of the most extensive nature—social, so called, political and religious—it cannot be fully discussed in this place. (Acland 105)

Acland takes for granted that these questions are social, and that social means the relation of the masses to (rather confusingly) "physical and moral causes." England claims to be civilized, but fails to act that way. The failure to recognize the interconnectedness of the whole community is what is implicitly barbarous: "The Community may be barbarous or civilized. We have here to do with Civilized Communities only. . . . I should be ashamed of dwelling on subjects of this kind, did I not feel that the People of England have yet to awake as from a dream. . . . We must feel the bitterness of the evil which social life entails on the less honourable members of the body politic" (105–07).

Having, in fact, already adverted to these "social" questions at some length, Acland disqualifies himself for further discussion and limits his following remarks to "most of what a Physician may venture to remark on the social condition of such a city as Oxford," to wit, "(1) Habitations; (2) Ventilation; (3) Drainage; (4) Medical care of the less affluent classes; (5) The relations between moral and physical well-being" (108), a broad set of categories indeed and one on which Acland actually has a great deal left to say, including recommending scientific and religious education for all and recreation in the arts, as "bad music" or "incorrect drawing" are "as great an intellectual evil as a foul smell is a physical one" (155). Here is the association of physical with moral fitness, and moral fitness with culture and the arts that will recur so frequently in the Parliamentary debates of the '60s on fitness for the franchise and will be the staples of John Ruskin's and Matthew Arnold's writings on the relations of culture and citizenship. The fifth category creates a site for Acland to insist on the value of the doctor's professional knowledge to diagnose public issues affecting all classes of society, and implicitly claims an authority equal to that of the clergy who had, up until the 1840s, dominated public conversation about the social meanings of cholera. Physical health is absolutely necessary to moral development, he argues, and, with education, is the primary concern of the medical profession and the state. Finally, "The main object of the State is assuredly to secure, as far as possible, the good conduct of the people" (Acland 149), for which good physical health, and the moral health that depends on it, is a prerequisite.

Acland was exemplary of a much broader phenomenon. By the '60s, the moral problems of inclusion in the social body were defined as problems of self-discipline through moral education, that is, socialization, which in turn was dependent upon providing an environment that would promote moral and cleanly habits. In short, public medicine could not be separated in this period from housing reform or from moral education. This burden fell heavily both on public health officials (to provide good sewerage and water quality) and on the domestic woman who was a primary target of sanitary education. She was to be responsible not only for the cleanliness of her home, but for the related moral and hygienic training of her husband and children. The housing movement itself, although legislatively concerned with sanitation—the destruction of slums, the repair of drains, the construction of new housing up to a certain code—was just as concerned (at the level of intervention) with the inculcation of proper domesticity, particularly among the lower working classes.

Although medics emphasized the need for expert knowledge to understand and treat epidemic disease, basic sanitary principles in domestic life were believed to be easily graspable, and appropriate for school materials, tracts, and other forms of propaganda. Falling into the domain of social education, and targeting a female audience, it is no surprise that sanitary outreach moved back into the purview of women and the clergy. A Ladies' Sanitary Association tract makes the analogy between home and body explicit:

> [Your skin is full of little invisible holes.] You will readily admit that three millions of holes and twenty-eight miles of pipes, are not likely to have been placed in the skin of a single body, without a purpose . . . they are DRAINS AND SEWERS WHICH THE GREAT BUILDER, WHO MADE THIS HOUSE FOR YOU TO DWELL IN, HAS FURNISHED for carrying waste matter away from it . . . *a quarter of an ounce of [decaying] poison is drained away* thorough the sewers of the skin, every day. (original emphasis, "The Use of Pure Water" 25–26)

It is said that clergyman and sanitarian Charles Kingsley, in visiting poor, sick parishioners, would carry an axe in order that he might begin his visit by improving ventilation in their bedrooms. The body, especially the body of the sick and impoverished patient, was like the "sick" house or slum—sanitary improvements must be structural. Like the "necessaries" installed at the order of the inspectors, good equipment had been given to the poor by God, but they failed to use it responsibly and care for it wisely.

The theme of overcrowding that already had become important in the '40s was central in the sanitary literature of the '60s. It was one of the knottiest problems for legislators. In 1866, member of Parliament H. A. Bruce warned, "The House had already dealt with two great causes of disease . . . [water and drainage of nuisances]. But the source of evil the most difficult of all . . . was the overcrowding of houses . . . in every large town thousands of persons were brought up in a state of moral degradation, which could only end in a great national danger" ("The Public Health Bill" 6). Individuality could not develop when the people were massed together as contiguous bodies. Medical science had also begun to insist on the importance of clean air, and the dangerous nature of air "vitiated" by previous breathing. Many medics determined the healthiness of a building primarily in terms of the number of cubic feet of air per person (ideally seven hundred). An underlying concern, however, in terms of "overcrowding" was not space but its uses. Housing historian Richard Rodger points out, "It was not simply the physical structures themselves which undermined decency and the family unit—there were many examples of generously proportioned and well maintained terrace housing and tenement flats—it was the congestion with which they were associated" (40–41). Descriptions of persons "of all sexes" huddled together in one room usually implicitly and often explicitly define incest as an inevitable result of such crowding.[19] "'Talk of morality!' [says Edward Bickersteth, in a lecture] . . . 'amongst people who herd—men, women, and children—together, with no regard of age or sex, in one narrow, confined apartment! You might as well talk of cleanliness in a sty, or of limpid purity in the contents of a cesspool . . . the first token of moral life is an attempt to migrate, as though by instinct of self-preservation, to some purer scene'" (quoted in Godwin, 21).

In turn, the city, and the population which is perceived as part of its structure, came to be seen as a large, unwieldy, and slovenly body, ever more in danger of dissolution.[20] Overcrowded central slums, corruption at the heart of the metropole, evoked suspicion, as did the city's extremities.

> Wide streets have been carried through the crowded haunts of the poor. But the population exists, and has increased. Thousands who did live in dark alleys are now driven to the suburbs, and spread over long, narrow, undrained streets. It is the *cincture* of a great city which is chiefly dangerous, and which often binds the population in a girdle of death. The barbarians that harass and threaten the frontiers of an extending empire are not more fatal . . . than the miserable, slovenly, uncared [sic] suburbs of a metropolis. (original emphasis, "Untitled")

The empire, with its diseased foreign climates, was a source of external dirt and corruption. Suspicion began to focus on the boundaries of the city—its skin, as it were—in addition to the long-standing concern with the dark and problematic interior.[21]

In viewing the "medical" and the clerical responses to the epidemic, one must keep in mind that the lines were not at all as clearly drawn as they appear: many medics were quite happy to believe that God had sent the pestilence and numerous clergy believed in the sanitary movement. Many of the early indictments of the clerical position were written from a sanitary perspective that was somewhat at odds with that of many professional medics. Finally, the sanitary position of moral environmentalism was not far off that of the clergy's notion that sin was the cause of disease—after all, for Chadwick, to be dirty *was* a sin. The similarities are probably best evidenced by the convergence of the two agendas in the third and fourth epidemic, under the rubric of "obeying God's Natural Laws." Other responses were clearly the result of a liberal or radical political agenda that not only favored scientific explanations but also resented the indictment of the poor and the reactionary religious intolerance of some clergy. However, these differences within the medical, sanitary, and religious positions did little to affect the sense of their presence in the public sphere, which was even by the second epidemic perceived as quite a bit more coherent and institutional than it actually was.

In the case of the church, the reasons for the initial apparent coherence of their position are fairly obvious. The cholera liturgy was official, and whatever some clergy might have thought of their brethren attacking the victims as sinners, they were hardly in a position to publicly denounce a position implied by the liturgy. The church, riven though it was, was still an institution, and an embattled one to which, with whatever private reservations, clergymen were publicly rallying. On the medical side, the evolution of a "public stance" was probably more accidental. Those who wrote at first may have been writing as outraged individuals, their use of a "national" rhetoric simply a result of having taken up the terms of debate offered by the church's rhetoric. Perhaps a desire to disassociate themselves from the elitism of the church—with which doctors had been lumped by working-class radicals in the first epidemic—may have motivated some medics to delineate their own position as well. Some writers were clearly self-identified as medics per se, others may have simply been sanitarians without medical training. Still, the widespread practice of basing the speaker's authority on scientific, positivist grounds that were the unifying factor for both medics and sanitarians, and the fact of sanitary institutionalization, made the discourse of such writers seem both coherently and officially medical. As the period progressed, the aleatory mobilization of nation as a legitimating discourse gave way to more purposeful and focused uses of the nation and social body concepts as a platform for professionalization and public service.

Regardless of the motives of the original writers, or of how they understood their intervention, this debate marked a significant shift in the medical community's representation as a public profession. First, it was the first time that medics (outside of the Board of Health) routinely directly addressed the public (in organs like the *Times* instead of addressing each other in medical journals) from a position of professional interest in and responsibility for the general weal. However they viewed themselves, their rhetoric situated them as members of a profession (sometimes in their pseudonym, sometimes in the text itself), whose expertise gave them the right—and obligation—to speak with authority, as those concerned with public, national issues. In the eyes of the general public, medics suddenly had a communal presence as policy arbiters and a (superficially coherent) position on those issues with which they could be identified.[22]

Sanitary issues were to remain the main platform for medics to involve themselves in public affairs, and by the mid-century, sanitation was becoming quite thoroughly medicalized, making medics much more central to the sanitary project. Through the sanitary movement, individual medics could have public medical careers, and the whole profession could have representation as the guardians of important governmental knowledges. Perhaps as much as the early Boards of Health, this public spat between a few medical writers and a dignified authority such as the church did much to legitimate medics as proponents of a scientific perspective and as a public profession. In any case, medics pressed the advantage. Earlier medical writers wrote for the general public on private issues—although the advice might have been good for a population, it was intended to be taken on a private level by an individual reader. Now medics began to write books for the general public that dealt with public policy issues, and gave advice meant to affect whole populations. The homogenization of the profession was to take many more years (assuming that one believes it has been achieved today—one might look at nursing to see most clearly that the legacy of status divisiveness lingers on, along with the linkage of lower status to the task of ministering to bodily needs). But the medical profession thus early on achieved a degree of coherence in the public sphere—that is, in the eyes of the general reading public—at least on the issue of public health, however vicious their internecine squabbling. In part, this apparent unanimity may have resulted from the relative unassailability of their position. Just as the sin = cholera equations of the church could not be challenged easily by other clergy in the public sphere, relatively few medics were willing to attack the sanitarians—who would want to come out in favor of filth? Also, although many medics offered contradictory opinions to the general public on the best treatment of the new and baffling disease, or on its contagious or noncontagious nature, that was quite different than implicitly attacking the position of the Board of Health, a duly constituted authority.

In Part I, I observed that sermons were constructed invoking two sets of shared knowledges: religious doctrine and current events. Nation became a mediating term between those two shared paradigms, and a term with some difficulty of definition. Medical explanations directed at the public relied on two different strategies: first, that of the sanitarians, whose goal, largely achieved by the '50s, was to make the sanitary idea as widely understood as Christian doctrine and therefore as compelling in explanatory power for the masses. The second, which gained force over the development of a culture of medical professionalism and specialization, was to impress the public with an exclusive scientific expertise. In this strategy, it was not important that the public understand *why* the epidemic should be interpreted in a particular way, but that the public believe implicitly in the knowledge of the medics who were themselves to construct its meaning, leaving the public to trust their oracular instructions. This approach was directed most successfully at other middle-class professionals and policy makers who respected science and believed in scientific authority. In both cases, attacks on religious interpretations did not so much offer a coherent alternative explanation, which would have been difficult given the utter lack of medical consensus, as they rested on a critique of clerics' unscientific attitudes and political conservatism. Such discourses relied on the exclusive nature of professional knowledge. Nation, as a symbol of the common ground of professionals and the public to which they minister, was most effectively mobilized by medics toward the end of the period, from a position of professional identification with government and an ethos of social service that legitimated their inclusion in public regulatory practices.

5

The Body in Question

IN THE DEVELOPMENT OF DISCOURSES surrounding the four epidemics of cholera in England, a number of complex issues were defined and contested. Crucial to many of these discussions were definitions of the body—individual, social, national, gendered, and classed. The discourses of the body in this period of time were multiple and fragmented. Their development cannot be narrated simply as a progression; their movement was erratic and often recursive. However, it is possible to compare these discourses at these temporal points and find that the visions of the body that dominated in the late 1860s did differ from those of earlier periods. The development of a powerful, officially authorized discourse on the body that emerged through state medicine's relation to cholera and the developments of the discourses "from below" that countered those formulations led to ways of thinking about the body that became central to modernity. These included competing perceptions of the body as surface versus depth and inscription versus essence, as well as problems of body management contested within the changing structures of power/knowledge.

The development of the medical vision of the body over this period moved in two directions: the first did not significantly differ from views widely held early in the century, relying on a theoretical understanding of the body as multiple systems—mostly intake and excretion, and to a lesser extent, chemical systems—which required balance to be healthy. Although incorporating new material and perspectives, this vision was not incompatible with earlier ways of thinking physiology. The second direction had to do with the emerging medico-surgical vision of the body, in which there was increasing attention to structures and seats of disease. Although the second set of views came to be dominant within medical professional writing, the sanitary perspective was still shaped by a general and fairly easily grasped notion of the body as systemically regulated by intake and excretion, especially through respiration. This view was compatible with popularizations of the new understanding of the body as always dying, always death producing in all of its processes. The theories of French physician, pathologist, and anatomist Marie François Xavier Bichat (1771–1802) were already becoming widely popular in Europe in the years after his initial influential publications in 1800–1801. Bichat insisted that clinical training should be paired with autopsies and postmortem examination of tissues. His ideas became well known in England through the mid-century as generations of surgeons trained in morbid anatomy in France brought back his views and disseminated them in England. Bichat theorized that life existed at two levels, the "animal" life of the whole organism and the composite organic life of its many tissues, which were continually dying and regenerating. It was this tissue-level life that most interested Bichat, who identified tissue as the basic unit of life and defined life as the sum of forces resisting death. In mid- to late-nineteenth-century British medicine, this view harmonized with new evolutionary theories of survival of the fittest. As popular medical discourses sought to harmonize these ways of envisioning the body, three trends emerged in sanitary literature especially, quite dramatically in the 1860s: a flattening of the body into surface; the emergence of a tendency to view the body's multiple systems (respiratory, alimentary) as having differences in substance (tissue) more important than differences of overall function; and an overriding concern with bodily output. Intake was characterized less in terms of type and quantity than of purity, and the ability to rid the body of—and distance it from—its excreta became a matter of urgency.

The beginning of the period posited a body that was, in itself, healthy as long as it was balanced, using an economic model focusing on intake of "fuel" to power the body without overstraining its ability to digest. The later model was one in which the body is essentially unhealthy—death creating, death infested. The essential task of health was to excrete that poisonous or degenerate—literally, decaying—material as quickly as possible. The earlier model is exemplified in the Society for the Diffusion of Useful Knowledge's (SDUK) 1832 instructions to the working man regarding the cholera and temperance: "if a man's natural spirits and strength are habitually exhausted by artificial stimulants, his stock of spirits and strength will be so taken up beforehand, that if the cholera makes a sudden demand upon this stock, even his life must go toward the payment" (160). To avoid "depleting one's stock," the reader is advised that

> Coarse sour food; spoiled vegetables . . . [etc.] are all unwholesome, and produce all the uneasinesses and evils of indigestion. Food that is too rich or too nutritious will produce the same kind of mischief, and even more whether it

happens to be digested or not: if not digested, just the same, and if digested, the additional mischief of plethora or fulness of blood, a state always attended with danger. . . . It is moderation that is everything. (164–65)

This point is repeated several times, and italicized at the end of the section. Moderate intake—neither too much nor too little, but just enough to keep all running properly—insured that a body was healthy and therefore resistant to external enemies. Later, however, the enemies of the body were most significantly internal. Whereas the body in the '30s was not itself dangerous to others, especially in health, by the '60s, the body was *essentially* dangerous—if it excreted healthily for itself, it poisoned the environment for contiguous bodies. As William Farr says, "Men . . . are always surrounded, in air and water, by an atmosphere of decaying matter, which is given off from their own bodies and from the animals by which they are surrounded" (*Vital Statistics* 166).

Cholera became a symbol of the persistence of this deathly and disgusting element within modernity. And, as such, cholera came to be associated with racial otherness, inappropriate femininity, immorality, intemperance, and filth. Yet cholera, in reminding Britons of the price of urbanization, also reminded them of the interdependent nature of the modern world. Economically, militarily, and geographically, it was not possible to contain the spread of cholera by simply withdrawing from contact with the outside world. Modern individual independence meant a communal interdependence in which space had to be shared, commodities needed to circulate, and exposure to disease could not simply be avoided. In this sense, the disgusting was indeed at the heart of civilization, not only as the guarantor of taboos but as the ineluctable proof of the human community's organic nature. Cholera was a constant reminder of the vulnerability of the interior of the individual body and the threat of that hidden interior surfacing—the eruption of a hidden filth onto the body's surface. The social body, like the individual body and its tissues, was essentially death producing, and never more so than in its rudest health.

MODELS OF CHOLERA

Throughout the period, medics were elaborating a plethora of theories about the nature of cholera. The first and most important opposition from the very beginning was between contagionists (those who believed the disease was propagated through direct human contact) and non-contagionists (who usually believed the disease arose from environmental causes)—a somewhat sloppy distinction embracing a host of positions much more complex than this binary can describe. However, this set of labels was used by the Victorians themselves, in part because it did capture the substance of an important division on the spectrum of beliefs about the disease. Margaret Pelling has admirably debunked the notion that most, let alone all, doctors were anti-contagionist, although sanitarians were so to some extent, perforce: if one is arguing that piles of dirt cause disease, one doesn't want to emphasize contagion as a source of illness. And, of course, strict contagionists were supposed to believe in quarantine, which was both anti-trade and medically old-fashioned. Many medics were some species of what has been described as "contingent contagionists," that is, they believed that other circumstances being right, cholera could *become* contagious. Such other circumstances included sanitary nuisances, or an "epidemic constitution" of the weather; in short, medics held a whole range of theories.[1]

If early on, the division between contagionists and anti-contagionist medics was already vexed, by the second epidemic, proliferating positions made that distinction extremely problematic, although sanitarians continued to uphold a public affirmation of anti-contagionism through 1849. Medics who believed in specific causes came up with a range of possibilities, the closest of which to germ theory (that is, the late nineteenth-century understanding that the disease was caused by a specific living disease agent) included William Budd's notion that "fungal bodies" propagated the disease and John Snow's theory that the disease was passed via the fecal-oral route through contaminated water. Those against contagionism cited high survival rates of doctors and nurses, although others disagreed.[2] Even in the 1860s, medics still frequently attributed cholera to atmospheric disturbances, electrical or otherwise. Many still believed in the venerable theory of miasma (disease spawned by bad air, often emerging from rotting material) and spoke of a bluish cholera mist that appeared before the epidemic began.[3] William Farr's influential "zymotic" theories of the 1840s built on the belief that decomposing matter was always noxious, which included the less obvious corollary that most things that were noxious were decomposing. This theory held that it was decomposing matter that causes cholera (among other epidemic diseases) by a kind of fermentation that made previously harmless substances dangerous. As late as the late 1860s, it was frequently claimed that cholera evacuations were not harmful until they had decomposed for several hours, at which time they became potent to cause illness.[4] Farr's work, essentially sanitary in its emphasis on the removal of decomposing materials, also accommodated John Snow's conclusions by provided for waterborne infection through decaying matter in the water supply.

In 1855, apothecary, surgeon, and physician John Snow had dramatically demonstrated the waterborne nature of cholera, removing the handle of the Broad Street pump in St. James's Parish, where contaminated water had caused a major outbreak of cholera. Even long after Snow's famous demonstration, however, most medics assimilated Snow's theory into an additive, "multiple causes," contingent-contagionist model.[5] Anti-contagionists also pointed out that if people thought it was contagious, fear of the disease (which was also thought to *cause* the disease) would get out of hand, to which Snow replied:

> British people would not desert their friends or relatives in illness, though they should incur danger by attending to them; but the truth is, that to look on cholera as a "catching" disease, which one may avoid by a few simple precautions, is a much less discouraging doctrine than that which supposes it to depend on some mysterious state of the atmosphere in which we are all of us immersed and obliged to breathe. (*On the Mode* 135)

Physician John Grove, in his pamphlet on the treatment of cholera by sulphur, attacked dogmatic sanitarians' character assassinations of their patients, complaining, "the non-contagionist harps upon 'propagation by contact . . .' being unproved, and sets aside altogether other modes of propagation; and to such an extent is this carried, that cases difficult to square with his views are thus dismissed:—'She had committed some act of intemperance'" (10).

The second major controversy was about the nature of cholera: was it a local disease seated in the intestines? Many thought this was impossible—a disease that wreaked such total havoc was clearly systemic, probably febrile in nature. Some sought a local pathology that would account for the gross systemic derangement, often by locating it in the nervous system. The logic of some of these attributions can be seen in physician and medical textbook writer Archibald Billing's discussion of cholera, before and after actually seeing it in practice. In 1831, Billing's two-page discussion of cholera, of which no London doctor had yet acquired experience, rehearses the common wisdom and positions it within his own nosology as a non-febrile disease. He recommends "opium, laudanum and brandy with hot water, hot vapour or water baths, and fomentations" (121), to counteract the weakness caused by purging. In the latter stage of collapse, he recommends stimulants and (unfortunately) bleeding.[6] By the fifth edition of his textbook in 1849, however, Billing's remarks on cholera are much more detailed, running in toto from pages 249–61, and he deems it a febrile disease, though he acknowledged that to some, this might "seem a startling assertion" (250).[7] Fevers, in Billing's model, do not result directly from external stimuli (although the possibility of an epidemic constitution of the atmosphere is still admitted), but from a lack of nervous force. In 1880, physician and textbook writer John Syer Bristowe still argued in his *The Theory and Practice of Medicine* that cholera had to be systemic, against claims that it was a local bowel irritant, because "foetuses of mothers dying of cholera themselves give clear indications of being affected with the disease" (223).[8] Cholera is listed here as a febrile disease. These discussions were among the most typical of attempts to pin down the nature of cholera; however, there was apparently no category of possible illnesses and no imaginable treatment that was left unexplored. Literally hundreds of books, pamphlets, articles, and chapters were devoted to cholera.

Cholera's mortality rate ran at approximately fifty percent, which became slightly higher with the unintentionally damaging medical treatment favored in the early part of the century. These treatments primarily involved bleeding, though even more drastic measures were sometimes used—cautery of the spine to galvanize the nerves, red hot irons on the skin to cause reaction against the cold caused by circulatory collapse, heated enemas, and so forth.[9] Brandy and other stimulants were much employed. Although desperate medics did attempt what would now seem the logical step of intravenous saline rehydration, the technique was neither antiseptic nor mechanically sound, and poor patient response discouraged this mode of therapy. Opium, as a common treatment for diarrhea, became the later treatment of choice, mercifully, although still often in conjunction with bleeding. Overall, however, an astonishing number of different treatments were used to no avail.

Treatment diversity reflected the wide range of theories about the constitution and seat of the disease, and of course, the sheer desperation of medics. Bloodletters who could get little blood from dehydrated patients cut all the more avidly under the belief that the answer to the lack of circulation was to restore the blood's liquidity by forcing it to flow. Those who believed cholera was a nervous disorder treated the nerves, whether with stimulants or sedatives; those who believed it was a fever tried either to foster the fever's "crisis" or to retard its progress, depending on the apparent strength of their patients. Even in the '60s, postmortems sought evidence of cholera's attack on the sympathetic nervous system. And as much, or perhaps more than the evidence of morbid anatomy, theories reflected the training and specialization of the medics who propounded them. Older physicians sought cholera in imbalance of the total system, whereas the younger generation of surgically trained medics hunted for the specific site that was its lair.

MEDICAL MODELS OF THE BODY THROUGH THE MID-CENTURY

Medical textbooks from the 1830s to 1870s demonstrate the development of this tension between "systemic" and "local" diseases—that is, between the integrative model of physic and the site-specific model favored by surgery—clearly and dramatically. In order to trace a mainstream trend in the organization of medical knowledge of the body in this period, I surveyed books that positioned themselves as introductions to medicine as a field, most of which were identified by their authors as targeting students and junior practitioners as their primary audience. All that I chose were written by prominent physicians, widely circulated, and went through multiple editions. In each, I looked at earlier and later editions to see what, if any, significant changes took place. Not surprisingly, they record increasing interest in pathology, in a more locally based or "surgical" view over a purely systemic view associated with the "old" physic, and toward treating diseases, both practically and nosologically, as separate, or at least separable, entities rather than as subtle gradations in the expression of systemic imbalance. (Perhaps more surprisingly, all showed a sudden shift toward addressing sex, race, and age as significant categories around mid-century, which had not been considered significant before.) In order to provide an easily accessible overview of changes in the organization of knowledge, I here provide comparisons of the texts' structure and excerpts from the introductions. The development of the period toward specialization and toward a tissue-centered vision of the body can be clearly seen through this simple comparison.

Archibald Billing's popular 1831 book, *First Principles of Medicine*, lays out a centrist position that accounts both for physic and the new emphasis on pathology.[10] He frames his book thus:

> The first step toward treating disease successfully, is to ascertain as far as possible, the nature of the *alteration* which has taken place in the *seat* of the *disease*, or what has been technically called the *proximate cause*; in default of this knowledge which is sometimes unattainable, we can depend only on analogies, drawn from what we know to be the fact in other cases, and from *physiology*, which is a careful *observation* of the *phenomena* resulting from the *functions* of the different *parts in health*. (his emphasis, 1831, 1)

This covers both bases. He goes on to acknowledge the need for the study of anatomy—after, and supplemental to, a course of lectures on the healthy physiology.[11] Despite a gesture toward the study of pathology, however, he ultimately divides up the body in only four systems: "the apparatus which supports the life of man . . . [consists of] the stomach and intestinal canal called the PRIMAE VIAE, the ABSORBENT VESSELS, the HEART and BLOOD VESSELS, and the NERVES" (2). This division indicates the plan of the book. He goes on to discuss the uses of stimulants and narcotics, and so forth, but there are no sections, simply a continuous essay. There is no discussion of special pathology—individual diseases are always discussed as various phases and intensities of general disruptions. In this first edition, the entire book was 131 pages. By the fifth edition of 1849, however, Billing was forced to defend his choice to have no table of contents—which he did by referring to the unity of the body as an organism and the inadvisability of dividing it into separate components. The introduction still followed the old structure, though with more detail, but the book ran to 332 pages.

But Billing's old-fashioned physician's emphasis on the unity of the body and relative downplaying of pathology, with its reliance on specificity and compartmentalization, had already lost favor with many readers, even by the 1830s. George Gregory offers a good example of the transition.[12] His popular new textbook, published at roughly the same time (the fourth edition appeared in 1835), was positioned as an update of William Cullen's 1785 work, still using Cullen's basic nosology, which had been dominant in the profession since the mid-eighteenth century, and directed to "students and junior practitioners." Nosological identification of diseases was crucial because treatment would depend on the proper categorization of the illness. Cullen's great work identified four major categories: the pyrexiae, or febrile diseases (including fevers and eruptive diseases like measles); the neuroses, or nervous diseases (including apoplexy and tetanus, for example); the cachexiae, or diseases arising from bad habits (including elephantiasis and scrofula); and the locales, or local diseases (such as cancer and anorexia). Gregory identifies four areas of new knowledge, one of which includes the two "new diseases," cholera and yellow fever.[13] His text clearly shows the influence (and emerging market appeal) of Bichat's theories and of the study of morbid anatomy. Gregory acknowledges new interest in epidemic disease, an area of knowledge that had not advanced much in England since the work of the famous physician Thomas Sydenham (1624–1689) until the cholera years. Gregory divides his 674 pages into two major categories of disease: acute diseases (including fevers) and chronic diseases. The acute diseases are basically systemic, under the classic model of physic, and the chronic diseases are those that have an anatomical seat (except for a small "chronic constitutional" category).[14]

Gregory's introduction is a masterful balancing of the surgeon's and physician's approaches. Although he categorizes systemic diseases "which fall under the particular cognizance of the Physician" as those that include fever or not, are acute or chronic, he notes that "A third distinction, equally elementary, is into constitutional and local diseases;—into those, namely, in which the whole system equally partakes, and those which depend, more obviously and immediately upon the laesion [*sic*] of some particular organ" (1835, 2). Having made this concession to the domain of anatomy, he quickly insists that these distinctions are "artificial boundaries" that serve as "beacons" for the diagnosis—but disease is, he insists, really more complicated and less categorizable than that: "It is, in fact, a most important principle in Pathology, that an intimate connection is established between all the parts of the living system, which must necessarily baffle every attempt to give a perfect idea of diseases by *separate* investigations" (his emphasis, 1835, 2). As a physician, he emphasizes the systemic nature even of "special" pathologies:

Diseases . . . have their points of *analogy* as well as of *dissimilarity*; and it is an object of consequence to determine these analogies, to show the great features of resemblance which all diseases bear, and to trace the almost insensible gradations by which they run into each other, and which enable us, whether to view them as separate objects of inquiry, or as the closely connected members of a great family. (1835, 3)

Yet, Gregory is not averse to keeping up with the times. By the sixth edition of 1846, twenty-five years later, the organization of the volume changed radically. Capitulating nearly completely to the increasing tendency to compartmentalize and specialize, the introduction states, "The pathologist . . . can trace . . . [in disease] many common features. . . . Still the number of distinct and well-defined diseases to which man is subject is very large, and the principle object of this work will be to describe them, so that they may readily be distinguished" (1846, 1). For vaguely defined diseases, he argues, pathology is the only answer to get at the truth of disease, and he is clear that there are two kinds: general pathology (physic) and special pathology ("seat" based descriptions of specific diseases and their effects). Cullen's classic nosology of disease has meanwhile been completely discarded in the previous edition, and Gregory adds here a section on vital statistics, showing just how much Farr had made the Office of the Registrar-General central to the medical profession.

Gregory explains that, as is generally accepted in this period, his "Special Pathology is limited to the elucidation of such complaints as have acquired specific denominations and are comprised under one or other of the fourteen general conditions of disease" (1846, 5). Although he retains his original systemic distinctions (febrile or not, acute or chronic, and so forth), he has now organized the book by "part of the body which principally suffers during their progress" (1846, 5), indicating a capitulation to a medico-surgical approach, even though, he warns, "All diseases are, in strict language, constitutional . . . all nosological arrangements of diseases, therefore, are artificial . . . and apt to mislead" (1846, 5). This volume displays the cutting-edge emphasis on medical and vital statistics and also on diseases specific to hot countries; London medics were starting to pay attention to colonial medics' experiences with the new disease threats and also to tropical medicine as a nascent field. At this time, some medical "textbooks" mention a tendency in the profession to deny that there is any such thing as "systemic" disease (although this is here referred to as an extreme position), whereas earlier it had been common to insist that there was no such thing as a wholly local disease, though of course lesions might only manifest in one locality.

Detailed though it was, Gregory's work seems to have been subsequently superseded in popularity by much more frankly compartmentalized works such as what would become an industry standard, James Russell Reynolds's *A System of Medicine* (1866).[15] This text unapologetically recognizes special pathology as its primary focus, to such an extent that instead of a unified text, the five volume set is largely a compilation of articles, each written by an expert on the particular malady. Of the labored and careful distinctions between general and special pathology that so deeply concerned his predecessors, Reynolds is dismissive in his relatively brief introduction: "The distinction between general and local symptoms need not detain us, since the terms are obvious in their meaning, and the difference between them is gradually dying out by the recognition of the fact that no one organ can have its functions or its structure changed without the existence of some relative change in all the rest" (1866, 13–14). The reversal is subtle but telling—instead of assuming a general illness that expresses itself locally, he offers a brusque acknowledgment that any local illness will have some "relative" effect on the rest of the body.[16]

This book also illustrates the emerging trend of presenting sex as a difference extending beyond reproductive structure:

> Sex cannot be said, accurately, to be a cause of disease . . . yet, in all modern treatises on medicine, it figures in the chapter on aetiology. . . . Several organs, and even systems of organs, present sexual distinctions although not forming part of the special reproductive apparatus. Not merely are such differences seen in the nervous endowments, physical, animal, intellectual, moral and emotional, but in the skin, the muscles and the bones. (Reynolds 1866, 9)

The third edition of *A System of Medicine* in 1876 showed few changes, and subsequent nineteenth-century medical textbooks continued the trend already in place without displaying any more basic epistemological shifts, though special pathology became ever more elaborate. John Syer Bristowe's *The Theory and Practice of Medicine* (1880), for example, has general pathology on pages 1–116; special pathology takes up the whopping remainder—pages 117–1136. Structure and function as significant distinctions are "generally accepted," according to Bristowe, and, although he laments perfunctorily that good organization is nearly impossible, he explains that he has grouped diseases by the descriptors "specific febrile" and "local" "with more or less disregard of accuracy" in favor of utility (ix). He proceeds with a tissue-theory approach deriving from Bichat's popular work on morbid anatomy, in which the systems of the body are based on types of tissue and their ceaseless individual cycles of growth, reproduction, and decay. For example, he subdivides his text, in part, as follows:

A. Properties and development of protoplasm.
B. Simple tissues—1, epithelial; 2, connective; 3, tubular; 4, organs
C. Development, growth and maintenance of the organism. Functions: 1, of circulatory system; 2, of digestive system; 3, of excretory system; 4, of nervous system.
D. Decay and death essential elements in the processes of life. (table of contents)

The real news here is that the text no longer begins with the whole body as a system, or even with systems of organs by structural function (digestive, circulatory), but by sub-tissue material (protoplasm), then tissue type (epithelial, connective), and finally to the systems of the whole body. This vision works from the microstructure up—from the fabric of life to the workings of the body. There is an increasing emphasis on cell biology and on death and decay as elements of life, as the capstone and overarching conclusion is the emphasis on death as integral to life.

Bichat's theories, already fairly widely disseminated in Britain much earlier in the century, were becoming fully institutionalized in the late '50s, and by the '60s were clearly incorporated into basic medical textbooks. Thomas Tanner's popular *The Practice of Medicine*, in its sixth edition in 1869, begins with a short section on general diseases, then proceeds by "system" subdivided by organ. He doesn't waste much time justifying his organization, but in his first section (under "General Diseases: Diseases of the Blood") frames the body this way: "The characteristics of the living organism are ceaseless change and ceaseless waste. Directly man begins to live, he begins to die" (1). Again, the tissue (blood) is prior in importance to the circulatory system, and death is accorded coeval status with life itself. Later books tended to emphasize cell biology and the constant feeding and wastage of cells and organs in their introductions. There was also much more emphasis on chemistry and microscopic examination than in earlier ones. In short, in the mid-century, the body is reframed again, not just as systems of organs, but as systems of structures made up of the very stuff of life, proto- or cytoplasm, which itself conducted a mysterious and constant process of decay and rebirth, of intake and especially of excretion. Tanner emphasizes, "There is an immense difference—a difference of life and death—between the blood which enters, and that which issues from, the lungs" (3). This formulation ran throughout the rhetoric of '60s' sanitary reform, with its near hysterical insistence on clean air and obsession with the wastes exuded in the body's respiration and perspiration.

Paradoxically, medicine had spiraled—from the purely systemic vision of the whole organism common to pre-pathological medicine of the mid-eighteenth century (with its moral-personal touch) through the emphasis on organs and macrostructures of the early nineteenth century, to an emphasis on microstructures of cytology and chemistry. These new foci were popularized as powerfully seductive and relatively easily grasped systemic models for understanding the body by reformulation within the terms of a Galenic notion of humoral homeostatic regulation that had never really fallen from popular favor.[17] However, instead of focusing on balancing intake, as did earlier models, newer representations of health posed the problem as one of the body's continuing efforts to rid itself of the deathly and poisonous substances engendered by its constantly decaying cells. Homeostasis, in this model, is achieved through the constant distancing of harmful body products from the body that produces them. All bodies, even healthy ones, were dangerous, constantly exuding death to be incautiously taken in by others, whereas the unhealthy body poisoned itself as well as others with its inability to properly excrete. In short, in addition to the move from old-fashioned physic to a medico-surgical view of the body that has been widely discussed, there was an institutionalization of the new emphasis on cytology and on racial and sexual differences concomitant with a predictable insistence on special pathology. With this came a model of a sort of biological thanotism, a death drive in the body itself. As William Farr put it, the "human body has a tendency to death" (*Vital Statistics* 216).

THE FILTHY BODY AND CHOLERA

The emphasis on the body as intrinsically disease producing seems a strange development, when one considers that medical science had a much clearer notion of how external agents resulted in disease in the '60s than in the '30s. One might expect that the '30s, with its notion that any tipping of the delicate balance of the body resulted in the generation of disease, would see the body as more intrinsically dangerous than later models that saw disease as invasive. In fact, as medical knowledge moved toward germ theory (as the theory that disease was caused by specific living organisms later came to be called after Louis Pasteur's discoveries in the late 1870s), popular medical discourse seemed to compensate with an ever-intensifying suspicion of the body itself. Early sanitarians wanted to clean acquired dirt off the body; later, they were concerned with cleaning the body's own perspiration off to keep the pores open for continuous excretion of the body's internally generated filth. The body itself was seen as filthy.

Historian and sociologist Norbert Elias has argued that the modern body emerges as a body concerned with closure of its openings and regulation of ingresses and egresses. Sociologist Pierre Bourdieu has also traced the emergence of the middle-class body, especially that of the petit bourgeois, as a body concerned with "narrowness," regulation and the diminution of excess. Certainly the gendering of the body, during the emergence of the rhetoric of separate spheres and the consequent reclassification (and re-anatomization) of female (and less obviously male) sexuality, confirmed this increasing focus on the disciplining of the body's openings.[18] This was particularly true of the body Bakhtin describes as the grotesque body celebrated in carnival—a body defined by its openness, especially of the lower body, its incontinence, in short, its publicness and impropriety. The grotesque body was increasingly identified with improper femininity or indiscriminate sexuality, pauperism, drunkenness, and the foreign (and, secondarily, with the decadent aristocracy). It is this body that was envisioned in polemics directed at legislating control of the body, and it is the "abject" products of this body, including disease, that had to be eliminated from public view. By the end of the 1860s, the ideal body was male, English, imperial, closed, and active. It was mobile, and its motion was outward; it was productive, rather than receptive.

Sanitary writings and other popularizations of medical models in this period tended to focus on the surface of the body as a dangerous point of contact between self and not-self. The most important tissue was that membrane that both divided and connected inside and outside, in mediated communication. Sir Alfred Power's 1871 pamphlet, *Sanitary Rhymes: Personal Precautions against Cholera and All Kinds of Fever*, intended to be educational for working-class readers, conveyed current medical understandings of sanitation and the body in verse, beginning, significantly, with "The Skin" (the entire body is summarized in three poems on the skin, the blood, and the nervous system, all tissues that mediate communication between the body and its environment).

> There's a skin without and a skin within,
> A covering skin and a lining skin;
> But the skin within is the skin without
> Doubled inwards and carried completely throughout.
>
> The palate, the nostrils, the windpipe and throat,
> Are all of them lined with this inner coat;
> Which through every part is made to extend—
> Lungs, liver and bowels, from end to end.
>
> The outside skin is a marvellous plan
> For exuding the dregs of the flesh of man;
> While the inner extracts from the food and the air
> What is needed the waste in his flesh to repair . . .

Verses follow on proper food, water, and hygiene. The poem concludes:

> All you, who thus kindly take care of your skin,
> And attend to its wants without and within,
> Never of Cholera need have any fears,
> And your skin may last you a hundred years!

(Power)

The body has become flattened out into a two-dimensional surface—a skin—in which the inside and outside of the body are not really differentiated as is the difference between that body and its environment. Instead of eating being a taking of materials inside through an opening of the body, through a clearly demarcated boundary between outside and inside, it becomes a placing-in-contiguity of certain, potentially dangerous (impure) materials with the porous surface of the body. The body is thus, in one sense, sealed (it has no openings, only a continuous skin). Even materials taken into the body are outside this skin (the stomach becomes a space exterior to the body proper), yet radically permeable (the whole surface is now a potential place of ingress and egress). Systems that would earlier have needed separate accounting, such as the digestive system, can be absorbed under this model. Eating becomes a form of respiration, just as breathing is tissue nourishment.

Cholera, of course, is quintessentially grotesque. The body voids itself of its digestive contents uncontrollably and frequently, in appalling quantity. Early on, the presence of cholera meant that the body had not been properly managed in its intake and output; by the '60s, it was readable as a body that had inappropriately taken in the most abject of materials, human feces. Attempts to recover "cleaner," more appropriate body materials were frustrated; venesection failed to obtain much material, and what could be obtained was "corrupt," "black," and "grumous."[19] Psychoanalytic theorist Julia Kristeva argues that abjection and the response to "abject" bodily wastes relates to their imaginal relationship with death; the body abject is the body dying, and the corpse is the final abject material. Cholera's tendency to turn the body "blue" or "black," the lividity and coldness of the body before death and corpselike shrinking of the facial features and extremities mimicked death in life; perhaps more horrifying to many was its tendency to upset the established markers of the boundary between life and death from the other side of the line. As Delaporte observes, "This singular pathology took on what had hitherto been death's surest and most stable features. Life was mimicking its opposite" (43).

Cholera corpses often seemed to *gain* heat after death, particularly in the abdominal region, and muscular spasms caused pronounced movement in the limbs and sometimes in the trunk for some time after death.[20] In their *Reports on the Epidemic Cholera: Drawn Up at the Desire of the Cholera Committee of the Royal College of Physicians*, physicians William Baly and William W. Gull assert that "Amongst the phenomena presented by the body after death from Cholera, are the well-known contractions of the muscles, which often occur to so great an extent, and last for so long a period, as to excite horror in the ignorant, and add in such minds a further mystery to this disease" (8). Additionally, they note, the temperature of the body, so cold before death, often warmed afterward. Since putrefaction often slowed after severe dehydration, also, there were many reasons to fear that cholera corpses were being committed prematurely to the grave. Indeed, these symptoms, combined with the Board of Health's insistence on quick burial fed popular fears that victims were being buried alive.

Cholera thus dramatized all of the anxieties about bodily control that mark humans' physical initiation into culture as "civilized" bodies, and singled out precisely those evidences of unregenerate physicality that mid-Victorian culture abjured. It is not accidental that, although cholera is not a sexual disease, the descriptions of the physical-moral environment that focused on filth conflated clogged drains with sexual license in the promiscuous overcrowding of the slums. Interestingly, almost none of the writings on cholera (except in case studies) mentioned the most dramatic feature of the disease—the copious voiding of the bowels, generally onto the bedding. The cramps, a secondary symptom, were instead used to define the disease—descriptions of people "taken" with the cholera often focused on images of people screaming, doubling over, or collapsing instead. The description of cholera "taking someone" suddenly, in the street or some other public place had tremendous currency throughout all the epidemics. Another prevalent narrative was that of cholera *foudroyant* (sudden and severe) or cholera *sicca* (dry) in which there was no diarrhea, but merely sudden collapse, unconsciousness, and death in minutes or hours, made more dramatic by the absolute health of the patient up until the moment of collapse. This image persisted throughout the period, and there was active debate between doctors as to whether or not cholera sicca existed. There are postmortems that list it as the cause of death, and note serous matter in the bowels, even though it had not been voided. Current knowledge of cholera suggests that such a pathology is physically unlikely. The fact that this narrative was so persistent, with its image of sudden and public attack and its suppression of the unpleasant but characteristic symptom is telling, perhaps, both of Victorian distaste for such details but also of the Victorian perception that cholera was not merely a diarrheal disease.[21] In essence, for public portrayals of cholera, the most salient symptoms seem to have been uncontrollable muscle spasms, the characteristic cyanotic color, and desiccated appearance—the abjection of a recently healthy (white) body into its unrecognizable opposite.[22]

Cholera, in short, was disgusting. As critic Winfried Menninghaus points out in his epic study, *Disgust: The Theory and History of a Strong Sensation*, by the late eighteenth century, philosophers had a carefully elaborated theory of disgust as part of their thorough analysis of aesthetics: "Eighteenth-century aesthetics discovered the basis for pleasure in 'unpleasant sensations' in their self-reflective dimension for the soul. . . . In its violent defense against the approach of something inassimilable, the unpleasant disgust-sensation evokes a particularly intense awareness of self. For nothing less is at stake in disgust than the physical or moral integrity of those who feel it" (357). Disgust, comprised both of repulsion and fascination, is persistently associated in Western culture with death, old age, and the feminine, with proscribed sexuality, fecundity, and the openings of the body. In eighteenth-century European aesthetics articulated around classical ideals of the body, Menninghaus points out, an ideal of the seamless, closed body emerged: as Herder put it, the beautiful body was like "softly blown" glass—a continuous line without interruption (quoted in Menninghaus 52). Openings of the body, and their implied relation to the interior depths of corporeality, were inherently disgusting, and had to be handled artistically with the utmost care in order to preserve the aesthetic experience. These theories continued to be foundational for nineteenth-century aesthetics of the body. Late-modern theories of the good and the beautiful were founded in opposition to the disgusting, and for such twentieth-century theorists as Sigmund Freud and Georges Battaille, civilization is, in a sense, founded *on* the disgusting—the inexcludable exclusion from polite intercourse, the organic real at the heart of social artifice. Modernity—and England considered itself to be at the height of modern progress—is based in part on the aggregation of bodies in cities and factories. At the same time, modern civilization, with its ideals of cleanliness and privacy, depends on the closure and isolation of clean bodies, separated from each other and especially their wastes: sewage and corpses being the ultimate disgusting materials. Cholera, especially after Snow's waterborne theory gained currency, was the epitome of a disgusting disease—caused by feces taken in through the mouth, causing the body to leak more feces in turn, and finally converting the apparently healthy body into a cadaver in a matter of hours.

The recognition of death at the core of vitality and of barbarism at the center of modernity heralded a new vision of the social body. Disease, and its exposure of the disgusting, needy, vulnerable body, was being recognized as the darker side of progress—not something to be exorcised through progress, but progress's shadow. The unprecedented vulnerability implied by the "socialism of the microbe," as American medic Cyrus Edson was to call it in the 1890s, inspired a revulsion of respectable society from the perceived medical threat of the poor. By the fourth epidemic, the population became a unity; Snow's theory, finally gaining in acceptance, highlighted the vulnerability of the social body and the urban corpus to invasion by its own wastes. The poor became not simply the victims of their own vice to be pitied or despised, but also enemies within. Once they had to be acknowledged as part of the social body, they became simultaneously more dangerous, more liable to be seen as foreign—wastes that had been expelled, yet reinvaded the body. The poor were figured as both foreign and feminized as the body itself became the fully realized modern body caught between its striving for closure and self-containment and its mortal openness and need. The poor represented the scandalous and barbaric persistence of disease, ignorance, and want at the core of the clean and proper modern state. The ideal individual and social body, then, was defined by states of dangerous permeability and dependence and the quest for impermeability and independence. Surgical and histological models of the body undergirded the sense of the population's dangerous continuity.

It is unsurprising then, as Britain increasingly came to confront its uneasy position as sometimes mentor, sometimes exploiter, and hostile occupier of its colonies, that the colonial situation would be read through lenses similar to those applied to problems of poverty and exploitation at home (just as the poor, the foreign, and women in Britain were frequently read through racial and colonial discourses derived from the colonial relation). Cholera itself was aggressively defined as an "Indian" disease, attacking a white population. By the fourth epidemic, the clergy had returned to the issue of individual guilt and readiness for salvation, and had largely abandoned the issue of national unity. Intervention in the progress of the disease was now entirely a medical concern. However, medical discourse was now doing the work religious discourse began—that is, to use a public rhetoric to weld the populace into a national unity with a common set of concerns. By the fourth epidemic, cholera was insistently racialized in medical discourse. Racial thinking had swept Europe at this point, and Britain in particular was beginning to take a racist turn in response to specific challenges emerging in the empire, especially the Indian Mutiny/Rebellion of 1857. And of course, disease generally had long been associated with the characteristics of the other. The next chapter will explore the colonial history of cholera—the quintessential colonial disease—and specific racial and gender entailments in medical discussions of cholera in the 1860s.

6

Race, Gender, and Cholera

AS MEDICS SHIFTED FOCUS from individuals to populations, the profile of patients vulnerable to certain diseases came to be based less on individual behaviors and more on traits thought to be innate and widely shared. Interest in race increased both with contemporary scientific theories and with augmented medical experience in colonial areas. Early attempts to classify the population afflicted by cholera emphasized class, occupation, temperance of personal habits, diet immediately preceding attack, age, and sex. Environmental factors included ozone level, temperature, prevailing wind conditions, weather activity, odor, elevation, among others. All of these factors continued to be of interest throughout the epidemics, but two major shifts occur in the mid-century. A new emphasis on race emerged, most strongly in the fourth epidemic. An increased emphasis on sex, with a reading of females as more susceptible to disease, began in the third epidemic and continued strong through the fourth. Medical writing on cholera exemplified how this new focus on "essential" biological differences intersected with the symbolic significance of the disease. Despite repeated findings that race and sex were not statistically significant, obsessive attention to these characteristics surfaced consistently in the medical literature of the period.

Race, hitherto an unimportant factor in epidemiological accounts, now became an indispensable category. Even those who had nothing to note about race stated that fact, implying the expectation on the part of readers that there *ought* to be something to say. Race, sometimes coterminous with what we would designate ethnicity, was also used to make clear physiological distinctions between healthy individuals in new ways. For example, in the second epidemic, the poor diet of poverty-stricken Irish compared to that of middle-class English was blamed for their high death rates. By the late 1860s, however, at least some medical professionals believed that the

Irish were constitutionally suited to a diet of potatoes, as suggested in this "sanitary rhyme" printed for the education and edification of the working-class public:

> Which is best of these foods will depend on the place
> Where the man is to live, on his Climate and Race;
> In some Tropical countries prime beef bears no price,
> Whole Nations subsisting on lentils and rice.
>
> Oh! Erin, prolific abode of mankind,
> Good nurse of the body, good nurse of the mind,
> How well dost thou fashion brain, muscle and bone
> Out of buttermilk, meal and potatoes alone!
>
> (Power)

The "Child of Europe!" on the other hand, is cautioned to eat from all the food groups. In short, instead of a universal male body that was implicitly northern European, and really just Anglo-Saxon, bodies were differentiated by sex, class, and race, all of which have also, as I will discuss, a gendered component.

RACE, GEOGRAPHY, AND CHOLERA: 1832–1867

One might expect that there would be less focus on gross characteristics such as gender and race during a period of medical specialization that focused on cytology, micropathology, and chemistry, rather than, as previously, gross lesions of structure. Once again, instead, medicine moved in the other direction. Earlier, I argued that medicine began seeing the body as intrinsically illness-producing just as research was identifying more clearly the external causes of disease. Likewise, just as medicine focused more intensely on the least obviously sexually or racially differentiated structures and substances of the body, there was a new insistence on the significance of such differences. In part, this may have been compensatory emphasis—sexual and racial differences did not have to be so accentuated if they were obvious, but had to be insisted upon when, in tissue under the microscope, they were in danger of being missed and forgotten. Certainly also, there were political and cultural reasons that might explain some of the emphasis on race and sex: new property laws; Britain's imperial activities. And of course, there were scientific reasons, stemming most obviously from Darwin's work on degeneration and sexual selection. For my purposes here, however, it is enough to note the fact of this new interest, and trace some of its discursive investments.

The 1866 cholera epidemic in England, in comparison to the preceding ones of 1832, 1849–1850 and 1854–1855, was marked by a significant shift in medical discourse regarding racial biology, as evidenced in official sanitary and autopsy reports, medical journals, and scholarly monographs. This shift was linked to new concerns about gender that surfaced in tandem with new racial theories. These materials show changing attitudes toward colonial subjects of other races and also the racialization of the British poor through degeneration theories. Racial theories were intricately related to gender, especially the feminization of the "emotional," "irrational" people of India, itself seen as a land that caused effeminacy and degeneracy in its people, and the construction of women as a site of imperial vulnerability.

Although medics had traced the geographical progress of the disease even in the first epidemic of 1832, there was initially surprisingly little geographical "blaming." In part because disease was not thought of as being caused by a specific entity, nor were diseases themselves necessarily particularized, medics were less likely to look to a disease's geographical origins than at its manifestations in the communities they were treating. In the first half of the century, although some argued this was the disease seen in India and traceable in its progress from East to West, there was a good deal of debate about whether "Asiatic" cholera wasn't really just a virulent strain of "English cholera" or autumnal diarrhea. Cholera was graced with many modifiers, the most frequent being morbus, spasmodica, or asphyxia. By the third epidemic (1854–1855), it was generally agreed to have originated in and to be endemic to India, but emphasis was still on the European version. A widely quoted *Lancet* article suggested that the modifier "Asiatic" should be dropped, since the disease was so strongly entrenched in England and should be studied in its manifestations specific to that area. To the extent that the disease spread in London, the "filthy" parishes of the East and South were largely to be held responsible. However, by 1866, the disease was referred to almost exclusively as Asiatic or Indian cholera, and the emphasis in medical writing was insistent; in 1867, the *Quarterly Review* reported at the conclusion of the International Sanitary Conference that "the whole odium of being cholera producers has been thrown on our Indian possessions" (Whittaker 16). At the same time, descriptions of the "filthy" parishes began to situate them in an imaginary Other to England—a "heathen" country submerged under and concealed within the otherwise healthy English metropolitan heart of Empire.

Strikingly, although race had been a significant part of epidemiological writings in the United States since at least the Yellow Fever epidemics of the century's early years, there had been little crossover of that emphasis into British writings on epidemic disease. After the mid-century, that changed radically. Race became an indispensable category in epidemiological accounts, and was more heavily biologized than before—though it still remained a slippery combination of biology, ethnic heritage, and geographic location. Geography and culture were still thought by many to change biology itself, which might then in turn become heritable; others were moving toward a notion of absolute racial differences that were located in the body and ultimately independent of culture or geography, even though perhaps initially formed by them in the distant past. Even those medical writers who had nothing to note about race stated that fact, implying the expectation on the part of their readers that there *ought* to be something to say. Geography and vulnerability to disease were closely related; Dr. John Parkin, in his 1866 edition of *The Antidotal Treatment of the Epidemic Cholera*, notes, "Although enjoying an almost complete exemption from fever—the endemic of his country—he [the "negro"] is more than usually susceptible of other diseases, when, by removal or other causes, he is brought within the sphere of their operation . . . the negro is peculiarly predisposed to the operation of the cause, whatever that may be, productive of the Epidemic Cholera" (270–71). Perhaps as an expression of Britain's ambivalent relationship to its imperial holdings, cholera comes to be seen in the light, quite specifically, of an invader from India.[1] Fueled by fears that the disease might become endemic to England if it had a chance to settle in "the subsoil"—in other words, that it might colonize British land—British authorities focused on the desirability of controling cholera at its site of production: a move that meant controling the behaviors and land of Indians, which were supposed to produce it.

Some medics attributed India's endemicity entirely to cultural factors. George Johnson, M.D., in an address to a missionary group, locates the site of production in Indian social practices, especially bathing in the Ganges. He describes these bathing practices as involving bathers' immersing clothing and bodies in water and also taking water into their mouths, then spitting it out for the use of other bathers. He continues, "we may reasonably hope that the time is not far distant when the natives of India may learn that the only sure preventive of cholera is through cleanliness in their persons, their dwellings, their food, and above all in their drink . . . [or] the scourge of cholera will continually recur" (26–27). Here we have the mid-nineteenth century rhetoric of the liberal state, also evident in the contemporaneous reform debates, in which pedagogic intervention can inculcate appropriate behavior in a population that transforms problematic individuals into manageable, clean, and proper bodies.

Others, however, took a more essentialist view. Susceptibility to cholera was biological, and although it could be mitigated by social intervention, such mitigation needed to be made with an eye to essential racial differences. Such strategies more directly involved the control of the problematic body, by placing within in a cordon sanitaire, for example. John MacPherson, in a tract entitled *Cholera in Its Home, with a Sketch of the Pathology and Treatment of the*

Disease, also locates cholera in India: "The idea has been broached that we should endeavor to stamp out cholera in its birthplace—that if we are to strike at the root of the disease, we must attack it in its home" (138). This, however, he declares impossible because of the nature and scope of the problem; cholera is inextricably entwined in the colonial landscape.[2] It is important to keep in mind that race, for Victorian thinkers, was more mutable and less tied to a biologically essentialist view than it has been in popular twentieth-century thought—geography was thought to have physical effects that were definable as racial—which is why Indian-born English children were often thought to be not quite English. Racial degeneration was a threat emerging not only from cultural or ethnic difference, but from the land itself. Race was tied to the geography that both produced it and limited its potential.

Although many attitudes can be found throughout the period, there is a developmental arc wherein the preponderance of views shifted from a more constructionist perspective, in which Indian land and peoples are seen as in need of colonial guidance to improve their situation, but not as substantially different in kind from the urban British poor (an outlook prevalent in the first part of the century), to a view of Indians as fundamentally biologically different (and inferior).[3] Alan Bewell notes that in the early nineteenth century, British slums and factories were often described as tropicalized environments that both foster disease and are similar to colonial settings (49, 270, and passim). However, by the mid-century, the environment of India was seen as essentially different from that of Britain and also as essentially productive of disease (Bewell 245). Although Mark Harrison points out that Anglo-Indian visions of India were much more nuanced, in Britain itself, India came to be viewed as a fairly simplistic and negative totality by mid-century: "guarded optimism about acclimatization and the colonization of India prior to 1800, gave way to pessimism and the alienation of Europeans from the Indian environment; a shift which was closely related to the emergence of ideas of race and the consolidation of colonial rule" (*Climates and Constitutions* 3).

Control of the social body through sanitary science became both a goal of liberal government and the measure of its success in this period. Control of disease was equated with civilization and Englishness, pitted against a threat of racial degeneration and social anarchy. Physician William Sanderson's indictment of Indian geography and social practice transitions smoothly into a discussion of disease among the poor of London—a landscape that can be reclaimed and a population that can be retrained. He remarks, "Cholera is known to have originated in India, which has long been well populated, even in the prehistoric period. Cholera could *originate* only in dense masses of population depositing excreta and other animalized matter over surfaces, from which it is carried by the percolation of the rainfall to the sources of the water supply" (his emphasis, 10). He quickly connects what he considers an irreme-diable situation in India with the threat that it will take hold in London's dirty "uncivilized" regions—which are reclaimable:

> [This proposal will] remove the foul blot, the most degrading and disgraceful state and condition of a portion of this the greatest and most wealthy city in the world; the metropolis of the greatest Empire! the centre of the commerce, the science, and the philanthropy of the world. The reclamation of East London has become an imperial necessity, and should be a national work; and before that necessity, vested interests should be compelled to give way. (iv)

East London here represents unacceptable otherness, analogous with colonial otherness, in the heart of the metropole. But this otherness is remediable, and therefore demands intervention. What cannot be helped in India is degrading and disgraceful when present in England.

BRITISH MEDICINE IN INDIA

It is important to understand the degree to which British national identity depended on India as an other against—and through—which to define itself. As Anne McClintock puts it, "Imperialism is not something that happened elsewhere. . . . Rather, imperialism and the invention of race were fundamental aspects of Western, industrial modernity. The invention of race in the urban metropoles . . . became central not only to the self-definition of the middle class but also to the policing of the 'dangerous classes'" (5). Britain's effect on India itself was enormous, and British activity was almost certainly at least partially responsible for the cholera epidemics themselves. Indians' actions, in turn, especially the events of 1857, shaped Britons' narratives of British identity, both cultural narratives of their Christian and imperial character and scientific narratives of the British body, just as did the world pandemic of a disease defined as "Indian."

Radhika Ramasubban observes that, following the war of 1857, vast numbers of British soldiers were sent to India. Previously one British soldier to eight native soldiers, the numbers were raised to attempt a one to three ratio (39). High death rates for these new soldiers led to some sanitary improvement for the remainder. David Arnold notes that one-third of British troop casualties after the mutiny were from cholera ("Cholera and Colonialism" 127). Vijay Prashad argues that the dominant European model of the modern state as the social body, already difficult in Europe to coordinate with classed and gendered individual bodies, did not work at all in India, conflicting with the "Manichaean" racial/colonial divide. Black bodies could not be mapped onto a European social body. A segregated society developed, of safe, relatively hygienic British communities set at a distance from "native towns" left to suffer unimproved sanitary conditions.

In 1861, Britain made its first systematic enquiry into sanitary conditions in Indian communities (Ramasubban 43). But sweeping and expensive changes were "beyond the brief of a colonial government. It took the pressure of the international embarrassment of being held responsible for the cholera pandemics by the International Sanitary Conference of 1866 (which decided that it was contagious, originated in Ganga and was spread by pilgrimage) to push the government to act" (Ramasubban 46). Still, even then they did comparatively little, according to Ramasubban, preferring to perfect segregation techniques (50–51). Ramasubban asserts that there was a growing public demand among Indians for sanitary control. The British government insisted that Indians resented such measures and were quick to see them as encroachments on religious freedom.[4] Whatever the reason, until the turn of the century the British government largely threw up their hands at the overwhelming task and allocated relatively few resources for it. According to Mark Harrison, most sanitary education offered by Britons in India was the result of private philanthropic work, and much of that did garner the approval and support of some Indian elites (*Public Health* 87–88). Although there were a number of local attempts to deal with sanitary improvement, these were limited in scope and faced complex political, cultural, and geographical obstacles.

International pressure in 1867 pushed the British government to attend to Indian health affairs, but the British were reluctant even to implement quarantine procedures related to Muslim pilgrimages that might alienate the Muslim community, at that time courted as an ally against the outspoken Hindu "middle classes" (Harrison 137). It was believed that interference with religious observance risked civil unrest. In 1869, the Punjab was given its own sanitary commissioner to advise the provincial government, but, as historian John Chandler Hume explains, his duties were impossible for one person:

> He was to advise the Punjab Government in public health matters generally. He was to investigate personally any unusual outbreak of disease. He was to visit all areas where "cholera fever, and similar diseases are epidemic or localized and propose means for removing them." Additionally, he was to devise a statistical system for the area and prepare several reports, as well as to be constantly traveling for inspections. (709–10)

The hapless soul who took on this task, A. C. C. de Renzy, proposed a system that would utilize *hakims*, the existing itinerant health care providers used by many Muslims, as combination sanitary inspectors and interim health-care providers in case of epidemic, while awaiting British medical assistance. This plan would, it was hoped, solve the manpower problem and also bring allopathy and native medicine closer together. Government killed the plan before it was tried (Hume 710–11).[5] His successor proposed a similar plan, with similar results (Hume 722–23).

Although British doctors in India borrowed heavily from Indian remedies early in the century, there was officially little respect for native health providers, and as the century progressed, the official British effort was directed toward winning them over to Western medicine whenever possible (Arnold, "Cholera" 136).[6] This follows the track of the writings on other Indian cultural practices, such as Hindu and Muslim bathing habits, which were in the Romantic period much admired as evidence of civilized cleanliness. By the mid-century, these habits were thought filthy and disease producing. At the beginning of the period, Indian medicine, like Indian hygiene, was considered somewhat venerable; by the mid-century, the British found little to admire.[7] As colonial medicine enabled colonialism to use "the body as the site for the construction of its own authority, legitimacy and control" (Arnold, *Colonizing* 8), the British came to regard the cholera that decimated white troops as a form of Indian counterattack on the Empire, justifying not only contempt for Indians' habits, but suspicion and hostility for the country and its population (Arnold, *Colonizing* 168–70).

Many historians have pointed out that epidemic cholera mortality in India (and worldwide) was at least partially a result of imperialism, although cholera was indeed a disease indigenous to India. Ira Klein argues that the combination of new economic conditions with the mobility they sponsored and, paradoxically, the extensive water transport systems constructed by the British, were responsible for much of the appalling rise in Indian death rates in the mid and late nineteenth century. For example, Klein refers to a "recorded toll of 22 million between 1887 and 1954" ("Imperialism" 492), whereas Arnold estimates at least 23 million from 1865–1947 ("Cholera" 120).[8] Modern transport systems facilitated the spread of disease (Klein, "Death in India" 640), and encouraged population movement, as did economic changes associated with modernization that depressed existing local economies (Klein, "Death" 645).[9] Cholera in the Punjab, for example, was a relatively infrequent threat until mid-century railroad expansion there escalated its depredations (Klein, *Imperialism* 506). Ralph Shlomowitz and Lance Brennan find that migrant agricultural labor for the tea gardens of Assam in the late 1850s sustained far higher cholera mortality than British troops traveling the same routes (326). They ascribe this disparity to poor sanitary conditions provided at the depots through which such laborers traveled and also to their poor physical condition (especially during famine years) and lack of immunity to the endemic diseases of the regions to which they traveled (328). The canals and waterways that were intended to help modernize India changed the land's ecosystem and caused flooding and contamination of drinking water sources.[10] Canals were built without corresponding construction of drainage systems (Klein, "Death" 649–50). These ecological and economic changes also, in some cases, contributed to problems of famine. Famine doubled and sometimes tripled the "normal" death rates of a cholera epidemic and also contributed to starting outbreaks by encouraging population movement and the consumption of "famine foods," as well as contributing to the debility that made individuals susceptible to infection (Arnold, "Social Crisis"). Sheldon Watts bitterly observes that engineers and medics are the two professional groups which most "contributed to the successes of the cholera vibrio" (201).[11]

Indian reaction to the epidemics, although rooted in traditions of the disease that predated the British presence, often interpreted these new disasters in terms of imperial invasion. In one situation, local residents believed that the cholera had struck because the British defiled a holy place by camping in it and then killing and eating sacred cattle (Arnold, "Cholera" 128). In another occurrence, British soldiers were believed to have "polluted" a holy well—in fact, a medically "correct" interpretation, since it was the soldiers who soiled it with cholera vibrios (Arnold, "Cholera" 128). In other cases, gods or goddesses were believed to be offended, either by the behavior of the British, or by the behavior of Indians affected by the British (Arnold, "Cholera" 128). Many Hindus considered cholera the manifestation of a deity, either a specific cholera deity, like Ola Bibi in Bengal, or a more general deity, like Kali, in a new manifestation (Arnold, "Cholera" 130–31).[12]

INDIA AND THE VIEW FROM BRITAIN

Britons, both in India and perhaps even more dramatically, in Britain, increasingly viewed Indians in terms of absolute alterity in the 1850s and '60s. From the eighteenth and early nineteenth century, when India and Indians were often respected as a basically healthy culture and environment that Europeans could adapt, or adapt to, India came to be imagined as essentially a site of filth and disease. Once a biological notion of race became popular, this tendency was only exacerbated. Although cholera had always been known to be from the East, this fact took on new significance as the disease was racialized. Thus, those Britons who succumbed to the disease and became its vectors were seen as subject to alien invasion, Easternized, not only by the disease but by vulnerability to it; in some sense, they were racial traitors through their orientalized bodies, which were culpably made so by neglect and/or weak-minded indulgence. As historian Vijay Prashad memorably puts it, Europe felt that its "superior government and climate were betrayed by a fifth column, the working class, which provided the disease with a door into the European body politic. . . . India, after 1832, became the 'natural home of cholera,' not to speak of disease generally, and India is the ultimate source of labour, the source of disease, in the dirty brown bodies of the colonized natives" (243).[13] Further, the land of India itself was seen as guilty of disease production. Whereas low-lying, damp areas in England were seen as unhealthy and vulnerable to colonization by disease, India, and the people and behaviors that were mapped onto the land were considered to constitute an ecological entity productive of evil.

Again, this reflects a change in European perception of India's climate from earlier times; as Harrison observes, Europeans saw the tropics in terms of extremes: paradise and hell. But as David Arnold has also discussed, there was a trajectory of emphasis, first on the heavenly side of the dichotomy, then, by the nineteenth century, solidly on the hellish end (*Problem of Nature*).[14] Arnold has also observed the tendency of many insular Britons to imagine the entire diverse geography of India as homogenously tropical (although Britons living in India maintained a rather more nuanced vision of the landscape, often one that privileged the highlands of India as quite salubrious). In fact, about half the territory sat above the Tropic of Cancer, including Bengal, that most tropical and dangerous of imagined places. Bengal was considered dangerous both in Britain (where many knew it largely as the home of cholera) and by British in India, (where it was considered among the most deleterious climates for Europeans). Bengali men were often vilified as the most deceitful, lazy, effeminate, yet bloodthirsty and sensual of Indians (see Harrison, *Climates and Constitutions* 47). Mrinalini Sinha has documented that, in the second half of the century, "manly Englishmen" often constructed themselves against the "effeminate Bengali," not least through contrast of Bengali and British treatment of women. As Macaulay infamously put it, "There never perhaps existed a people so thoroughly fitted by habit for a foreign yoke. . . . The physical organization of the Bengalee is feeble even to effeminacy. He lives in a constant vapour bath" (quoted in Sinha 15). (Note that his environment is responsible for his enfeebled state, but the word "habit" indicates his culpability for his own oppression.) The Bengali male was often described as effeminate and sometimes as feminized; that is, the Bengali male was sometimes seen as an inadequately masculine male, and sometimes seen as more directly *like* or comparable to a European woman (except that, as a male, his state was degenerate whereas the European woman's was normal). In turn, European women's reproductive abilities were considered especially susceptible to the effects of the tropics in this period (Harrison, *Climates* 50–51), in part because of the heat's supposed weakening of the nervous system.

In a tradition extending back to Hippocrates, landscape has often been held responsible for disease. With the attention paid to the "deleterious place" in England as sanitary science turned to housing and landscape improvement (drainage, elevation, sewerage), it is quite natural that the land and built environment would come under scrutiny, as it did in the housing movement of the mid-century. However, even more important than the actual geography of India was its geography as represented in the British imaginary. As Arnold demonstrates, "by the late nineteenth century, India's incorporation into the tropics was becoming increasingly evident. Its diseases, . . . agriculture, even its people, were steadily brought within the framework of tropicality . . . as, in part, a consequence of the growing authority of imperial science and the connections being made between several parts of the tropical empire" (*Problem* 171). In other words, economically and agriculturally, India was being assimilated into a geographical model that benefited the metropole.[15]

India's much maligned climate and "tropical" image itself became important for Indian nationalism (Arnold, *Problem* 184–87). Environmental images and symbols "have often been a powerful emotional rallying point and a focus for an emerging sense of national identity" (Arnold, *Problem* 185). However, they were equally important for *British* nationalism. Practically every text in which a Briton denounces Indian environment includes an explicit favorable comparison with Europe in general, and often Britain (or the northern countries) in particular. Indian "tropicality" was necessary for the anxious definition of Britain's difference, and usually, superiority. The British imagined Britain's landscape, by contrast to and through the lens of imagined representations of its colonies, and especially through "the jewel in the crown," India. Britons set their Christianity against Eastern "savage customs," British science against Indian "superstitions," and enlightened British gender relations in comparison to Indian zenanas and suttees.[16]

As early as the '30s, Moreau de Jonnes had made the connection between religious pilgrimages, troop movements, and cholera. Unlike in Europe, where anti-contagionists were strongly motivated to ignore this kind of transmission, this fact was publicized right away by Christian missionaries hostile to native religion (Arnold, "Cholera" 140).[17] By the 1866 International Sanitary Conference, troop movement was forgotten, and the horrendous mortality among coolie laborers moving to work in British-owned tea gardens was quietly overlooked as well; the conference proclaimed religious pilgrimage the single most important factor in transmission of the disease. Arnold notes, "The attack on cholera was also an assault on Hinduism, one which was all the more authoritative for its invocation of medical science . . . [and] made the pilgrims into a 'dangerous class' requiring special measures for their regulation and surveillance" ("Cholera" 141). In India, as well as in Europe, the poor and sick were most susceptible to cholera, a fact well known in India. In Britain, however, in the popular imagination, these class distinctions between Indians were probably less clear than the idea that, as Prashad puts it, Indians generally had dangerous "dirty brown bodies."

Especially after the rebellion of 1857, Britain's narrative of itself as the so-called "Aryan big brother" to a developing India changed in favor of a more dichotomous racial narrative of the white man carrying his Christian burden and the deceitful, sexually ambiguous, racially degenerate native. The movement of imperial desire for and fear of this native is traceable in countless travel articles, anthropological studies, and adventure stories. The twin tropes of exploration and (often sexual) conquest became dominant metaphors for understanding the colonial relationship. In this way the object of desire (and of the journey) was both made central and neutralized by the clinical discourse of the scientist/military administrator who was the colonial equivalent of the urban doctor/policeman. Nancy Aycock Metz points out that the literature of sanitary reform in Britain pointed in two rhetorical directions: the literature of exploration, with its "emerging cliche of 'deepest, darkest London'" and to sensation fiction, with its sense of hidden secrets in the midst of respectability (65). The lower classes and the indigenous populations of the colonies had much in common in terms of their roles in supporting the industrial capitalism of empire. These texts both othered the human and geographical objects of "clinical" interest and called attention to their proximity and centrality, their necessity to the reading subject. The expression of that double gesture was the invitation to the middle-class British reader to go on "expeditions"—to take "sanitary rambles," traversing distance while insisting to the reader that there is simultaneously no real distance involved. Both London and India were exhilarating sites of adventure and imperial masculine self-construction as a civilizing influence; both were also dangerous, sexually inviting, and representative of abject, inappropriate bodies that might strike the health of both the imperial individual and social body. Cholera was the Empire striking back, the colony colonizing the metropole.

Class, gender, and race were interimbricated with particular urgency in the late 1850s through the 1870s as Britain moved, not without trepidation, toward an officially Imperial identity. Following the revolt of popular British sentiment against Indian natives after the rebellion of 1857, and the uncertainty about Britain's role and responsibility for the events that preceded it and the appropriateness of Britain's subsequent responses, as well as other colonial expressions of discontent, such as the Fenian disturbances, gender and race stereotyping often mirrored each other. The gender stereotyping that Patrick Brantlinger traces in the British reaction to the Indians in *Rule of Darkness: British Literature and Imperialism, 1830–1914* can also be seen in relationship to Britain's own working classes in a period of reform legislation: the working class or colonial male was split into two types: one hypermasculine, sexually violent, uncontrollable, and bloodthirsty; the other, effeminized, sexually perverse, irrational, deceitful, and easily intimidated. The depredations of cholera measured the racial degeneracy of the population it struck.

The working classes in England also came increasingly to inhabit the position of the Other within the metropole, governed by a viceregency of middle-class cultural missionaries/police. At the same time, representations of relationships between genders and classes increasingly developed homologies with the colonial dynamic. In 1867, the *Quarterly Review*'s report on "The Cholera Conference" (the International Sanitary Conference) principally concerned itself with tracing the progress of the disease from various other locations, most notably India and the Mediterranean, to "the present year [in which] it has overrun the whole of the continent, and has attacked England" (Whittaker 30). Although the cholera was supposed to have come originally from India, many physicians believed that the disease lived in "the subsoil," and, if established long enough in a given new site, could get into its subsoil and thus, become endemic to the new location. The rest of the article evaluates the conference's recommendations for containment, using specifically military terminology, planning to "attack" the "enemy" "at a distance"—in the Red Sea, in fact (Whittaker 50).

Parliamentary records confirm this preoccupation with the "naturalization" of the cholera in Britain. The disease is described as an alien enemy from the colonial lands that attempts to "penetrate" and lodge itself in domestic soil. In the 1860s through the 1880s, when the appropriate role of the British civil servant was contested within an emerging awareness of and sympathy for the subjectivity of the colonial Other, the entanglement of the discourse of empire in the discourse of gender bears close scrutiny. The feminized and infantilized "Aryan little brother," for example, had to be reconciled with the hypermasculine Indian soldier of the still clearly remembered war of 1857, just as middle-class women were becoming disturbingly visible in traditionally masculine public spaces in the metropole.[18] The disruptive power of these changes was clearly visioned as a threat to Empire through the integrity of the imperial subject's masculinity. As Anne McClintock notes, concern about contagion was related to "boundary order" between races, classes, genders, which in turn "expressed intense anxieties about the fallibility of white male and imperial potency" (47).

Concern for cholera's invasion of Britain's subsoil was reflected in the fear that the heart of the metropole, "deepest, darkest London," was tropicalized. Alienated, inhabited by degenerated savages, moist, and filthy, these regions of Britain and their inhabitants, like the Indians, appeared habituated to dirt as if it were their natural element. Alan Bewell notes that the framing of cholera as a colonial disease was "not easily separated from the framing of the diseases of the urban poor, especially since that group was seen as the means by which the tropical or foreign diseases traveled into the very heart of the metropolitan city. The pathologizing of the urban working class occurred in tandem with the pathologizing of colonial peoples" (270).[19] Since they were

Britons (or at least that inferior species of Briton, the Irish), with a relatively small population of foreigners and Jews (not quite foreign, but certainly not considered English), their unfitness could only be explained through degeneration. And, like the Indians, or like Britons who lived in deleterious climates, these urban dwellers produced sickly, degenerate offspring. However, again because they were Britons, they could be saved, through what McClintock has called the "reversible" trope of progress/degeneration (43).

If the land was degenerate, causing degeneration of its people, it would in turn lead to further "racial" decay. As William Farr explains,

> the history of the nations on the Mediterranean, on the plains of the Euphrates and Tigris, the deltas of the Indus and the Ganges, and the rivers of China, exhibits this great fact—the gradual descent of races from the high lands, their establishment on the coasts in cities sustained and refreshed for a season by immigration from the interior; their degradation in successive generations under the influence of the unhealthy earth, and their final ruin, effacement, or subjugation by new races of conquerors. The causes that destroy individual men lay cities waste which in their nature are immortal, and silently undermine eternal empires. ("Influence of Elevation" 174)

Farr thus provides a neat justification for imperialism, as well as staking Britain's racial claims to leadership on its public health. Farr explains that the cholera is the warning, sent by God, that the British community is in danger of this elevation-related degeneration because so many have settled near the Thames: "the pestilence speaks to nations, in order that greater calamities than the death of the population may be averted. For to a nation of good and noble men Death, is a less evil than the Degradation of Race" (178). At the same time, descriptions of the "filthy" parishes began to situate them in an imaginary Other to England—a "heathen" country submerged under and concealed within the otherwise healthy English metropolitan heart of Empire.

CHOLERA, RACE, AND GENDER

Britons, then, constructed their national geographical identity in part against the tropical, colonial lands and peoples most meaningfully symbolized by India and Africa. They elaborated a national masculine gendered identity (here, English—after all, the Irish, or even Celtic peoples generally, were gendered ambiguously also) against the feminized or effeminate Indian male. The equation of the English woman with the Indian male made for awkwardness—certainly there was a *difference*, but a difference that could be elided rather easily. The British woman who transgressed, especially sexually, came perilously close through degeneration, to a native racial type. Sinha quotes British orientalist and politician Lepel Griffin, writing in 1892 on "The Place of Bengalis in Politics":

> The characteristics of women which disqualify them for public life and its responsibilities are inherent in their sex and are worthy of honour, for to be womanly is the highest praise for woman ... but when men, as the Bengalis are disqualified for political enfranchisement by the possession of essentially feminine characteristics, they must expect to be held in such contempt by stronger and braver races. (quoted in Sinha 35)

Herbert Sussman has suggested that British middle-class masculinity was predicated on the control of a "liquid, pulpy" sense of the undisciplined body and on the rigid control of desire.[20] I would argue that this liquidity is always already seen as feminine, the femaleness within the male that must be controlled to produce masculinity. If that liquidity and uncontrollable desire was projected onto the female and colonial male body, then cholera was the disease that most clearly symbolized that lack of control.

Associated with filth and intemperance of every kind, cholera symbolized loss of control of the boundaries of the civilized body and its most intimate secretions/excretions.[21] As the *Times* put it, "Dirt and debasement are convertible terms. That a man who is filthy in his person or his clothes shall rarely be sober is an almost necessary consequence" (Place Collection). The civilized body, like the civilized businessman, did not take in or expend its substance recklessly, and never allowed the boundaries between inside and outside, between life-giving substance and death-dealing excreta, to become confused. Imperial masculinity depended on self-regulation and controlled heterosexuality, as opposed to the warlike Northern Indians' or Arabs' homosexual practices or the Bengalis' too-luxurious uxoriousness. (Christopher Lane and Sara Suleri, among others, have documented the fascinations and terrors of imagined and real colonial homosexuality and homosociality for imperial Britons.) The cult of sport and gentlemanliness that arose among middle-class British men, especially those from whom colonial administrators were recruited, was focused on the redirection of male sexuality, in excess of appropriate fulfillment in marriage, through sport. The British administrator, deprived of traditional soldierly or working-class ways of demonstrating masculinity, displayed his masculinity through self-control and sportsmanship.[22]

Fear was not masculine and not English, and fear was, as early as 1832, blamed for causing cholera through a "hysterical" derangement of the body allied with other forms of intemperance: "To fast as well as to overload the stomach was equally pernicious. . . . Alarm . . . had of itself the power of exciting, not only hysterical sensations, imitative of the true disease, but the true disease itself. . . . Next in fact to errors of diet the depressing passions of the mind were perhaps the most frequent means of developing the choleric germ" (Gaulter 133). The temperance discourse linked the practice of intemperate consumption of alcohol associated with working-class males with other forms of intemperance and femininity. In 1832, the Society for the Diffusion of Useful Knowledge (SDUK) already described the conquest of cholera in terms of imperial character:

> [Cholera] is checked by [man's] skill and his firmness . . . it will finally be banished from the well-governed regions of the earth altogether. First, it will disappear from those which it has most recently attacked [England, not yet in the metropolis];—and, in the end, as the blessings of civilization extend themselves to every region on which the rain from heaven falls, or the sun of heaven shines; and as man improves in knowledge, virtue and power, and by degrees converts vast spaces now neglected into spots of fertility and happiness, and is himself raised in the scale of creation,—not the cholera only, but all the most severe febrile diseases, will probably be utterly banished from this globe. (202–03)

As disease spread inward toward the metropole from a degenerate periphery, health, through "man's firmness" would circulate outward throughout the social and imperial body.

The place of empire within the social body was subject to constant redefinition. It is certainly true that British attitudes toward colonial natives changed over time. The aforementioned optimistic excerpt is exemplary of an inclusive rhetoric modeled on the idea of the Roman Empire, wherein citizenship was an opportunity to be made available to those civilized individuals within "developing" communities. By the '60s, the attitude toward inclusion of the periphery in the social body tends much more toward the "Manichaean" one identified by Prashad, wherein the Indian body is the irredeemable abject. Progress, it seems, and even man's "firmness," carried one only so far. If the British imperial project lost faith in the viability of an imperial social body, it was all the more necessary to reinforce the boundaries between those firm (or at least potentially firm), closed British bodies that were progressing toward the "higher type" and the leaky, needy bodies of degenerating Others.

In addition to the emphasis on race, which is explainable within the discourses of Darwinist racial biology and racist reaction to the colonial disturbances of the later 1850s, there was a second, new focus, which was less clearly contextualized. This was a sudden interest in sex as an indicator of morbidity, with females being read as more susceptible to disease, which began in the third epidemic and became stronger in the fourth. The most dramatic evidence of this tendency is on official postmortem forms, in which a new column for reproductive organs suddenly appears. In summaries of postmortem examinations, "structural" change to the female reproductive organs is noted. Generally, it is agreed that "no change" is discernable in male reproductive organs—to the extent that no description of them is tabulated in collective postmortem descriptions (though female reproductive organs are described). In fact, it seems likely that male reproductive organs were rarely examined during cholera postmortems, since there was no call to describe them and medics expected to find nothing there. However, later descriptions suggest that certainly *some* traces of abnormality should have been evident in male genitals after a cholera death. Changes in female reproductive organs do surface in postmortem descriptions at about this time. This change had not been pointed out in the literature on earlier epidemics—possibly because of the relative lack of systematic postmortem exams of cholera victims, and possibly because doctors either were not looking carefully at the reproductive system or did not find significant pathology there (and I would like to stress this point, as the fact that the condition of the uterus in these postmortems, which seems to duplicate the appropriate condition of the uterus during a phase of menstruation, may be here suddenly pathologized). Perhaps it may have to do with the increasing use of the speculum at this time, which rendered a comparison with healthy uterine conditions more possible. In any case, this difference is at this time agreed by some medical writers to be worthy of note, although its significance remained unclear. By the fourth epidemic, it had become a widespread (though by no means universal) belief, largely unsubstantiated, that females were more vulnerable to cholera than males.

These structural changes generally consisted of irritation or discoloration of the mucous membranes and the presence of mucous discharge, sometimes discolored with what appeared to be blood. Interestingly, although physicians say they can come to no conclusions about the cholera from their examinations of reproductive tracts, they dutifully describe the appearance of the inner lining of the uterus, the fallopian tubes, and the inner labia:

> The mucous membrane of the labia becomes also inflamed. This is noticed in girls; the labia are red and swollen, and their mucous surface is covered with a pus like discharge. In women, a pink discharge, similar to that of the menstrual period, has been found; it lasted three days or more and ceased, w/out treatment. It has been noticed, in post-mortems on these cases, that the mucous membrane of the uterus is congested as if in the process of menstruation. (*Clinical Lectures* 459)

How this appearance would differ from a "healthy" uterus is not clear. There is no attempt to correlate patients' menstrual cycles with these observations; these patients may seem to be nearing menstruation because, in fact, they were. Or it is possible that illness precipitated a change to the cycle; from the data given, it is impossible to guess, and it is clear that these physicians did not ask that question. In any case, there is no baseline given for comparison to a healthy uterus, so that *any* description is framed as pathological.

Most peculiarly, in all of this emphasis on the female reproductive system, there is no provision for a statistical analysis of the effect of pregnancy on prognosis. In fact, in case after case, this is not even mentioned—and never included as part of the analysis of cases. There is no column for it on the returns. However, lecture notes at the London Hospital mention—with impressive documentation from cases under care there—that all pregnant patients admitted with cholera aborted. In reviewing case studies, it became evident to me that all patients advanced in pregnancy died, without exception, immediately before or after giving stillbirth (M'Carthy and Dove 448–49). The only other published mention I have found in surveying a considerable amount of the literature in English is in Baly and Gull, who state offhandedly that "It has often been stated that pregnancy is a predisposing condition to a fatal attack of the epidemic. Such an opinion is by some degree supported by the mortality at the child-bearing period"—that is, age 25–45 (155). They stress, however, that "Too much weight must not however be laid upon this fact," because mortality rates are generally higher for females in that age range and in the one immediately following.

If it had been often stated, it must have been in conversation—the mortality of gravid women had rarely been discussed in medical writings on cholera in English up until this period. One paragraph, which dismisses the possibility of a significant relationship, is all that is devoted to it in Baly and Gull's large tome.[23] This and a couple of other references are the only mentions of this important tendency in the large body of professional literature that I have surveyed. When mentioned at all, it is raised offhandedly as a curiosity, something unsubstantiated and not very important. Yet, judging from the London Hospital records, pregnancy had a significant bearing upon prognosis. The high rates of mortality there may well have to do with the fact that most people were advanced in the disease upon admission. Still, even in 1992, Barua and Greenough cite a fifty percent risk of fetal death in the last trimester, usually within twenty-four hours of the onset of illness, and also mention that placental retention is a common complication after miscarriage (21). Certainly the period is voluble on the subject of the delicacy of the pregnant woman's health; why then, would this not have been seen as worthy of analysis?

If femininity is the "marked term" here, what of the unmarked term? In other words, what does the examination of the male reproductive system show us? Generally medics agree that "no change" is discernible in male reproductive organs—to the extent that no description of them is tabulated in collective postmortem descriptions. In most cases, either the space under "reproductive" was simply left blank in the event of a male subject, or the column itself might be labeled "uterine tract." However, later descriptions that I found elsewhere suggest that abnormalities should have been evident in at least some male genitals after a cholera death, particularly a protracted one, if from nothing other than the effects of dehydration and circulatory collapse. There is mention of scrotal gangrene found in convalescent Indian male cholera patients (see Goodeve, in Reynolds). Indeed, a very early *Lancet* article describes cholera's usual effect on the appearance in male genitals: "the genital organs of the male are commonly purpled, the scrotum is wrinkled, and the testicles are drawn up to the ring" (Editors, *Lancet*).

Reproductive pathology seems to have been so clearly aligned with the female body that there simply appeared to be no point in looking at the male genitals. By the fourth epidemic, it had become a widely shared belief, largely without statistical foundation, that females were more vulnerable to cholera than males. Dr. Edwin Lankester remarks, "women are more subject to this disease, or it is more fatal to them than men. Of 145 fatal cases in Sunderland, 63 were males and 82 were females." The next sentence reads, "It appears that the black and coloured races of mankind are more predisposed to take the cholera and to die with it than the white races" (54–55).[24] The proximity of the two sentences register the apparently obvious connection, needing no transition, between gender and race as essential, and linked, categories.

The belief in sex-linked vulnerability is a particularly interesting development, since there is no historical justification for it from previous, fairly well-documented epidemics. It is a belief that arises somewhat mysteriously. Although in some districts, it is born out in small samples (e.g., in Wapping, significantly more women died than men), in most others, no significant difference is discernible. Baly and Gull's massive survey of the literature on cholera turns up one possible source in their entry on postmortem appearances of cholera patients. Under "Female sexual organs" (there is no entry for male) they note that Berlin pathologists Reinhardt and Leubuscher find structural changes of female organs common. They speak of the usual symptoms and a light "menstrual"-style discharge even in persons amenhorreac or post-menopausal. However, they also observe that the celebrated German physician Rudolf Virchow found no unusual condition in "the genital organs. . . . In women there was very commonly a menstrual . . . condition of the ovaries [and] extravasations under the peritoneal covering of the ovaries," causing them to look "mottled." Yet in contrast, the French researcher Emile Leudet is cited as having found nothing unusual in the female organs at all (Baly and Gull 57–58). Baly and Gull themselves find, in their thorough analysis, no correlation between sex and mortality, noting that although fewer females died than males, the numbers were closer than in most other maladies, wherein far more males usually died than females (154). India-based doctor Edward Goodeve, in his article on cholera for Reynolds' five-volume *System of Medicine* (1866), also comments on sex but only to say there is no effect.[25]

Examination of materials in the London Hospital archive reveals possible explanations that, though debated in medical circles, did not seem to filter down to the level of discourse addressed to the general public. The "Report on the Cases Treated in the Wapping District Cholera Hospital" found that of fifty-one males attacked, fifteen died and of sixty-six females attacked, thirty died:

> With regard to the class . . . nearly all were badly fed and worse housed. . . . The influence of sex might appear . . . to be more important than perhaps it really is. . . . The men, whose occupations are more laborious, take care to be better fed. . . . The man getting his chop where he works, while the wife and children sip their weak tea and eat bread and potatoes, with a little dripping or salt-butter, at home. (Woodman and Hickford 473)

Snow also comments on similar findings, quoting Farr on the effect of sex:

> at the beginning of the epidemic, the deaths of males exceeded the deaths of females very considerably . . . when the mortality from cholera attained a very high rate, the number of deaths among females exceeded the deaths among males. . . . The greater part of the female population remain almost constantly at home, and take their meals at home, whilst . . . men move about in following their occupations, and take both food and drink at a variety of places; consequently, in the early part of an epidemic, when the disease only exists in a few spots, the male part of the populations is most liable to come within the operation of the morbid poison . . . [later] it may reach those who stay at home as readily as those who move about; and in addition to the risk which the women share with the men, they have the additional one of being engaged in attending on the sick. It is a confirmation of this view that when the cholera poison is distributed through the pipes of a Water Company, the above rule does not hold good, but a contrary one prevails, owing, probably, to females being less in the habit of drinking beer than men, and being therefore more likely to drink water. . . . When the mortality of the whole of the metropolis during this period is taken together, there is a slight preponderance on the part of the males. (Snow, *On the Mode* 120)

Females may also have been less likely to be taken to the hospital early in the progress of disease, so that more were moribund at admission. The autopsy form in the report quoted here includes a column for the uterus but none for male reproductive organs. In an era in which femininity is aligned with racial otherness and the representation of vulnerability to forces that weaken social control, woman's body becomes a site of suspicion. Much like race, sex becomes a category about which it was expected there be something to say in the context of social control. Many scientifically informed medics, like Snow, dismissed such a connection, but by this point, sex and race had to be mentioned, even if simply to refute their importance.

This period also saw the passage of the infamous Contagious Diseases Acts. Driven by anxieties about the spread of venereal disease, especially in the military, the acts located the site of disease production in the genitals of women, specifically, female prostitutes, and set up a system for their forcible examination and therapeutic incarceration in lock hospitals. The rhetoric surrounding this discussion was fraught with images of racial degeneration and national insecurity (danger to the military), and was also widely extended within the colonial setting, as historian Philippa Levine has discussed in *Prostitution, Race, and Politics: Policing Venereal Disease in the British Empire*. My point here is simply to reiterate that there is in this period a tendency to locate danger, and often a specifically racial danger of degeneration, to the British social body in the reproductive system of the woman, institutionalizing the female genitals as a key site of epidemiological control. It is woman's difference that makes her weak, and also that makes her closer to the racial other— the Indian or the "negro." That difference is to be located in her sympathetic nervous system, so intimately dependent, according to the medical opinion of the day, upon her reproductive organs. In Germany, cholera, as a disease associated with degenerate physicality and loss of control over the body, "could only function as a term of abuse," as Evans observes (*Death* 230); in 1890s' Hamburg, it was associated with the "corrupting bacillus of Judaism" and foreign workers (400).

Medical textbooks before mid-century rarely had much to say about sex, surprisingly enough. In Gregory's 1846 medical textbook, for example, there is nothing on race or sex etiology. In the late '50s, however, that began to change, and sex, along with age, usually received some attention in the introduction to the volume. Exemplary, once again, is James Russell Reynolds's massive 1866 edition of *A System of Medicine*, which introduces the topic under the etiology section of the introduction under causes:

> Sex cannot be said, accurately, to be a cause of disease . . . yet, in all modern treatises on medicine, it figures in the chapter on aetiology. . . . Several organs, and even systems of organs, present sexual distinctions although not forming part of the special reproductive apparatus. Not merely are such differences seen in the nervous endowments, physical, animal, intellectual, moral and emotional, but in the skin, the muscles and the bones. (9)

This is quite different from earlier treatments, which, if they mentioned sex, tended to note that sex could only be considered significant in that it meant the presence of certain organs in a patient which could then be diseased (e.g., uterus, prostate).

As literary scholar Kate Flint has shown in a survey of several medical treatises, prevailing opinion at mid-century was that women's sympathetic nervous system (SNS), connected to her uterine system and her digestive tract, was more vulnerable than a man's to both mental and physical sense-impression. This is a discussion that became more heated in the 1860s and '70s, as women claimed more rights after the 1857 Divorce Law and as the debate about gender and education really got under way (see Flint 53–63 and passim). Those who were less rational and more emotional were of course more under the influence of the sympathetic nervous system, which was believed to be related to the digestive and reproductive organs, and influenced through them. Of course, if a woman's whole body was controlled by her reproductive organs, she must be particularly vulnerable to disorders affecting the sympathetic nerves. Thus, the feminine nervous system (also sometimes coded as incomplete or immature) should be more vulnerable than the masculine, the black more than the white, the "animalistic" laborer (or the effete dandy) more than the "rational" artisan or middle-class businessman, the intemperate more than the temperate. One debate at this point was whether cholera was a disease of the blood or of the SNS, as affected through the digestive tract—if of the SNS, then, given these assumptions, medics might indeed expect to see more female vulnerability to cholera, in the same way that racial "effeminacy" would similarly create vulnerability. Were cholera a disease of the blood, however, race and sex would have less impact.

Even as early as 1831, India-based surgeon Reginald Orton cites other studies to conclude that when the cholera was at Mauritius, even when many were not ill, "convulsive affections resembling hysteria were unusually frequent among the European and mulatto women belonging to the regiment" (450), and that it was chiefly prevalent among prostitutes in Bengal (455). There was a strong tradition of seeing "nervousness" as predisposing patients to epidemic disease, and "nervousness" was a feminine weakness. Once cholera was considered as possibly a nervous disease, such gendered references multiplied. John Chapman, physician and progressive publisher of the *Westminster Review*, made a strong argument for the cholera's attack on the SNS in a number of publications from 1865–1871. In his book on diarrheal diseases, in a chapter entitled "Diarrhoea Originated by the Mind," he gives several examples, all female, whose emotional stimulation brings on diarrhea, including this: "One of my patients, who was reading George Eliot's noble work 'Romola,' assured me that the emotions it excited in her brought on diarrhoea!

In fact, owing to this remarkable transformation of emotions into 'motions,' she was obliged for a time to abstain from reading the book" (4). He also gives some examples from the military, mentioning one very refined "gentleman" and "many soldiers, especially young ones" who have a similar reaction to fear, which upsets the sympathetic nervous system, causing diarrhea.[26]

Both Indian masculinity and the depredations of tropical diseases were seen as direct violations of this code of British masculine self-containment, a helpless dissolution of the male body into abject fluidity. Hence the emphasis on the questionable or immature masculinity of the young recruits whose fear deranges their sympathetic nervous system and thus their bowels, or the sentimental effect on the lady reading Eliot's *Romola*. It is the immature or insufficiently (racially) developed male who is subject to such humiliating losses of control, in the same way it is the drunkard or the gambler who has corrupted the healthy physical or economic system who is subject to infection—evidence of the persistence of eighteenth-century models of femininity as immaturity.

A flurry of other publications advanced this view of cholera. William Sedgwick's *On the Nature of Cholera as a Guide to Treatment* (1866) was "intended to illustrate the theory, which refers the disease to functional disorder of the central parts of the sympathetic nervous system, excited through the medium of the stomach" (iiv), and cites the suppression of urine without the accumulation of urea in cholera patients and also in hysterical females as evidence (61–77), although there is no reference to the morbid anatomy of the uterus. John Parkin's 1866 *The Antidotal Treatment of the Epidemic Cholera* also affirms that "This . . . is a disease which consists in the suspension of the organic functions—those functions over which the ganglionic [he specifies in a note that this means sympathetic] system of nerves presides," entering through the lungs (13). Thomas Giordani Wright, M.D., explains that it is accepted that "Secretion is a process of life by which the blood is converted into certain healthy products; and by affections of the sympathetic nerves, the secretions are altered in their nature. The only effect which we can conceive to be the result of a paralysis of those nerves, will be a conversion of the process of secretion into an exudation or elimination" (128). This explains why the liquid portion of the blood is converted into waste and excreted through the bowel.

Edward Goodeve's article, however, asserts that cholera "probably enters through respiratory or intestinal surfaces," affecting the blood, not the SNS. He also remarks both that sex has no effect (135) and that habits have "less influence . . . than has been supposed" (136). The habits of the underclass, particularly intemperance, dirtiness, and the general immorality with which these characteristics, and indeed poverty itself, were associated had long been blamed for their susceptibility to cholera, as poor neighborhoods were always hardest hit. It is these habits that were thought to make the British poor degenerate and animal-like, that is, comparable to inferior races. These debates obviously had implications both for racial theories of disease and for social policies bearing on disease control. If the disease was of the blood, then gender and racial characteristics were insignificant; if of the SNS, then these characteristics were crucial. However, in the very gesture that essentializes those characteristics, there is also the destabilizing possibility of degeneration. Between the apparently stable categories of blackness and whiteness, there is the British white underclass, especially the Irish, whose behavior can make them biologically like savages, but whose biological susceptibility can also be modified through behavioral intervention. Between the categories of masculinity and femininity there is similar slippage; perhaps there is little wonder that the search for a stable maker of difference might be sited in the apparently evident material reality of the uterus.

Altogether, what is one to make of the brief and apparently inconsequential appearance of the "dead end" investigation of sex- and race-linked cholera mortality in this period? The persistence of the belief in the significance of race or sex, against all empirical evidence—and against the pronouncements of many experts—is baffling from a strictly scientific point of view. There was almost literally no reason to believe that race or sex made much difference to cholera mortality. I would argue that it offers some illustration of both the extent to which what the "objective eye" sees is determined by cultural expectations and the extent to which, for example, the woman's body, especially the working-class woman's body, was racialized, pathologized and seen as key to biopolitical social control at mid-century. Policing the woman's body in this period was increasingly identified with preserving racial integrity, just as maintaining the domestic woman's appropriate presence in the home was increasingly identified as the precondition for the reproduction of the liberal subject. Efforts at sanitary and moral education in this period, for example, were particularly directed at women in their capacities as wives and mothers; on the other hand, the slovenly, intemperate, or sexually inappropriate woman was seen as especially dangerous (for the same phenomenon in Hamburg, see Evans 457–58). Working-class women's poor domestic habits were blamed for the social conditions that caused epidemics to spread, including the drinking of their husbands, which unbalanced the homeostasis of their masculine bodies and so feminized them. And of course it was precisely women who cleaned up after and took care of the sick who were most at risk of contagion; Richard Evans classifies cholera as, among German women, predominantly a disease of servants (458–63). Cholera victims, mostly working class or underclass throughout the period, were seen as degenerate and racially akin to the Indians who "produced" the disease. The domestic woman who produced the imperial male was thus a site of both strength and danger; her uterus, like the subsoil of the mother country was vulnerable to alien (germi)nations. In order to save English land from the fate of degeneracy—tropical disease becoming endemic in England's soil—problematic English bodies had to be saved from degeneration. To the extent that the disease was racialized, the key to its presence in England might be found in the weak link between the English and the racially Other—in the uterus of the degenerate woman.

Part III

Writing Nation's Body

It may be of comparatively little consequence how a man is governed from without, whilst everything depends upon how he governs himself from within. The greatest slave is not he who is ruled by a despot, great though that evil be, but he who is the thrall of his own moral ignorance, selfishness, and vice. Nations who are thus enslaved at heart cannot be freed by any mere changes of masters or of institutions.

—Samuel Smiles, *Self-Help*

> The humours of the peccant social wound
> All pressed out, poured down upon Pimlico
> Exasperating the unaccustomed air
> With hideous interfusion. You'd suppose
> A finished generation, dead of plague,
> Swept outward from their graves into the sun,
> The moil of death upon them.
> —Elizabeth Barrett Browning, *Aurora Leigh*

7

Narrating Cholera and Nation

THERE IS, ON THE FACE OF IT, a surprising dearth of direct literary response to the cholera. It is all but ignored in the Victorian novel, and almost never explicitly described. The Victorian penchant for avoiding names of diseases in print or describing symptoms, even in "realist" writing, until nearly the end of the century perhaps contributed to authors' discreet treatment of illness. Often, cholera, or something that might be cholera, shows up under the general euphemism of "fever," used widely by laypeople as a descriptor for all epidemic diseases, as well as a number of endemic ones. There was almost no novelistic treatment of cholera specifically in the earlier part of the century, with the exception of Harriet Martineau's *Deerbrook* (1839). Most novels that address it come after the '50s, and even then, there are not a vast number. Of the authors who do directly mention cholera, some merely name it in passing, like Trollope or Barrett Browning, and others use it largely as historical background, like Eliot in *Middlemarch* (1872)—though Eliot also provides a richly elaborated commentary on the general relation of the healthy body to the polis that I will discuss later. Novels that make it a central focus are few, published later in the century, and tend to be didactic—a Society for the Promotion of Christian Knowledge (SPCK) novel, *Through Tumult and Pestilence* (1886) by Emily Lawson, which I will discuss here briefly along with Charlotte Yonge's *The Three Brides* (1876). (Oddly, it emerges as a didactic topic after the last epidemic in the United Kingdom is long over.) A notable exception is Kingsley's 1857 novel *Two Years Ago*, which I shall explore in detail in the next chapter.[1] Drama of high enough pretensions to have registered with the Lord Chamberlain seems to have largely avoided it, for reasons that are perhaps obvious; and indeed, "fever"—a term that often encompassed cholera—could do the same ideological and symbolic work without the difficulties of stage representation or the unpleasantness of directly evoking an almost obscene disease in pages meant for the "Young Person."[2] Poetry, in addition to the ballads and doggerel discussed earlier, seems to have been the privileged venue, within which cholera could be easily personified and euphemized and actual symptoms elided. Of this literature, much was directed at a working-class audience. This material tended to advance a unified view of the medical and sanitary projects, and showed unsanitary conditions as a failure of hygienic habits among the poor. Material directed toward the middle classes used epidemic disease to indicate a more complex series of problems, usually including ignorance and bad habits among the poor, but also a failure of responsibility in the upper classes. Epidemic disease also provided the background for stories of the heroic (or, occasionally, not so heroic) doctor, and plots related to professional conflicts and development. But, as in political and church rhetoric, much of this material put cholera to work as a marker of class conflict and social failure. However, the novelistic form especially tended to emphasize solutions to do with culture and self-cultivation, rather than directly political or religious strategies of social therapy.

Scottish poet and songwriter Charles Mackay's "The Mowers: An Anticipation of the Cholera, 1848," was a typical example of the kind of cholera-themed poetry between the popular ballad and the didactic work. Less focused on a specific political question than on general moral issues, the poem still takes up the theme of the two nations in the metropolis. The poem begins with a gothic scene: three spectres, "Gaunt and tall and undefined," on one of the bridges of a great city, by implication London, on a foggy night. The city is "Huge, unshapely, overgrown / . . . Mammon is its chief and lord / . . . With Pomp and Luxury and Pride; / Who calls his large dominions theirs, / Nor dream a portion is Despair's." Each spectre speaks in turn—first, Suicide, who boasts that he is lord of the town. Drunkenness claims that his is pride of place, as suicide is the slayer of the "unit, I of the ten." Pestilence is the third; he exceeds their boasts, as he slays thousands "with a breath." Pestilence seems to represent disease generally, though he mentions typhus as one of his specific weapons. However, he points out, that the greatest "Lord of the crowded town" is one who is coming: Cholera. If men were wise, "they would not work for you, for me, / for him that cometh over the sea; / But they will not heed the warning voice. / The Cholera comes, rejoice, rejoice! / *He* shall be lord of the swarming town. / *And mow them down, and mow them down!*" (Mackay's emphasis).

Mackay targets poverty and vice and filth as related, though he doesn't eliminate the possibility of contagion either ("I brew disease in stagnant pools. / And wandering here disporting there, / Favored much by knaves and fools, / I poison streams, I taint the air"). He also uses a rhetoric that might be a gesture toward sanitarians' notions of overcrowding or Malthusian ideas about populations: cholera comes to help the first three spectres "thin this thick humanity," and the city is "teeming" (twice), "crowded," and "swarming."

These conditions are the result of human actions: men unwisely "work" for the spectres. But the most important sign of all that is wrong in the city is its poisoned, damp atmosphere. The first line of the poem reads, "Dense on the stream the vapours lay," and the spectres themselves are "built of mist and wind." In all this murkiness, we are introduced to the city: "fair to see . . . / Into its river, winding slow, / Thick and foul from shore to shore, / The vessels come, the vessels go, / And teeming lands their riches pour." Trade is a measure of the wealth of the imperial city, but it also brings foreign diseases; the miasma of the polluted river hangs over the entire city, as the river recurs throughout the poem. Suicide's victims drown in it, Pestilence's victims are the "main" to which all the dead in military disasters from Caesar and Alexander to Waterloo are by comparison, "but a river." (Again, the image of Britain as heir to world imperial lineages is invoked here.) Finally, cholera "cometh over the sea" in a watery apotheosis of destruction.[3] Mackay invokes the sanitary rhetoric of low-lying, damp ground, not only because he believes it to be scientifically correct, but because by the time he writes, his audience would have thoroughly internalized these sanitary ideas themselves. In its indictment of human agency and vice, rather than sanitary measures per se, it follows a tradition of such poems. Irish poet Michael Banim's 1831 "Chaunt of the Cholera," for example, alludes elliptically to the cause of the downtrodden throughout the poem, implying that "freedom" is the antidote for the cholera: "I kill for Freedom, / When Freedom wars with Might!" (4). The cholera here is personified as an ethical teacher who is brought "From my proper clime and subjects / In my hot and swarthy East, / North and westward I am coming / . . . And I come not until challenged, / Through your chilly lands to roam! — / As a bride ye marched to woo me, / And in triumph led me home!" (3). Banim, like other pro-Reform writers, borrows the logic of the church (the cholera is the hand of God) but also specifically politicizes it (God's vengeance is on oppressors, not Sabbath-breakers).

CHOLERA AND DIDACTIC NOVELS

Didactic novels for the poor tended to be more graphic than middle-class literature and to use cholera as an index of multiple sins, sanitary and otherwise. *Through Tumult and Pestilence: A Tale of the Bristol Riots and the Cholera Time* (1886), Emily M. Lawson's SPCK novel, is a cautionary tale that weaves together temperance, money management, and maternity with tales of the reform riots and the cholera. Annie, the young woman protagonist, is well meaning but thoughtless and weak willed. She marries Fred Harrison, the Adam Bede-like, stern, temperance hero, who ignores the worthier Mary for Annie's pretty face. Annie gets into debt buying clothes, and then fears to tell her husband, which damages his public character when she cannot pay household bills on time. Fred moves his family to another portion of town to save his child from the "river fogs," only to move inadvertently closer to bad drains and bad company. When he leaves Annie alone to work, she falls under the influence of her irresponsible cousins. She gossips and goes to the pub, becoming slatternly with the house and ignoring her baby, whose delicate constitution is undermined when he is frightened at being left alone. When the cholera comes, he is carried off first, and Annie becomes gravely ill, although she does recover sadder and wiser.

The link between drinking, fiscal irresponsibility, rebellion against authority, and death is further reinforced in a scene of the cholera riots, where looters too drunk to save themselves from a burning building are found dead, one clutching a bottle, the other a purse. Fred, however, who has saved a wealthy family's little son, while heroically ignoring his grandfather's patronizing insults, is suitably rewarded. The common humanity of rich and poor are asserted when both boys (both named Johnnie) die of cholera. Like Fred's Johnnie, the wealthy Johnnie's constitution is undermined by a fright—that of the riots.[4] Drinking and rebellion kill the children of rich and poor alike, through the common threat of cholera. Johnnie's mother, however, befriends Fred and his family, giving them a new cottage to live in, and Fred a much better job.

Writing for the working classes could apparently be a bit more forthcoming about physical details of illness than literature for a middle-class audience. Lawson writes that the "atmosphere of the house, where cholera had been doing its worst for eight hours, was so overpowering that Harrison felt momentarily sick and faint" (128). The narrator describes a cholera attack, wherein a sailor who has been drinking "gave a scream which rang down the quiet street, and doubled himself almost to the ground, clutching Harrison's arm as he did so" (105). Impressed, Fred thinks, "'I didn't think as it was so horrible. It must be a bad pain to make a strong man cry out like a whipped child'" (105). His wife's appearance shocks him and he fails to recognize her: "the corpse of a shrunken old woman it seemed, with livid skin, lips drawn back from the teeth, and eyes turned far up into the head" (113). The SPCK publications preferred simple and forceful language, not only for its impact, but because it was believed that such language was suitable to the level of the intended readership, and certainly it still fell far short of the bluntness of radical publications and entertaining broadsheets aimed at this audience.

Doctors are represented as sensible, practical men with the best interests of the people at heart, and interestingly, though the ministry is on the side of the medics, the curate is too delicate and nervous to be at the bedside of cholera patients. It is the lawyer who is most able to assist: professional men are the saviors and guides of the villagers in times of crisis. They enlist Fred to help them convince the backward, ignorant poor to vacate their cottages and camp on the common, away from the open sewer that is a source of pestilence. It is the poor who attribute the cholera to God, and insist on staying where they are, either out of habit or the sense that the pestilence is God's will, whereas the middle classes are represented as progressive and rational. Professional men are represented as the allies and structural analogues of the intelligent, temperate, skilled artisan, Fred—the ideal worker. He depends on them for direction and they depend on him to mobilize consent among members of his own class. None of the infighting between these authorities is represented, and indeed, they are represented as univocal, although frustrated by a lack of working solutions to the cholera problem.

In addition to the conversion of Annie and other survivors, cholera makes unlikely heroes of people who never catch it: a fallen woman is redeemed in her selfless nursing; scolding Clara becomes a caring and submissive wife to her "drunken brute of a husband" (thus managing to save his soul before his death) and concludes to Fred and Annie, "I'd never have learnt how good you were, or tried to be good myself, if it hadn't been for all the bitter troubles of the cholera time" (159). Fred's lesson is to become more paternal: less judgmental of those who fail to live up to his own high standards, and more willing to take responsibility for guiding them to better behavior. In short, he must become the link between the proper social body and those who remain just outside it, and that link is formulated in terms of his domestic role rather than a political one.

In middle-class novels, the doctor was also posed as a class mediator. Aimed at a higher-class audience than the SPCK novels, but likewise intended primarily as religious instruction, were Charlotte Mary Yonge's 1870s works. A devotee of John Keble and the Oxford movement, she wrote many novels and histories, including the wildly popular *Heir of Redclyffe*. Her 1876 novel *The Three Brides* shows the persistence of sanitary rhetoric long after the medical acceptance of Snow's model; in her novel, the filth and poverty of "Water Lane" bring about an epidemic. As is so often the case in her novels, however, sanitary insufficiency symbolizes the failure of the ruling class to act in a timely way. In *The Three Brides*, the ruling family, the Poynsett Charnocks, suffer illness and death within the family, mirroring the loss of life in the slum. Although the disease is described as "a fever," and its symptoms vary with different characters from lethargy to hallucinations, to a sore, swollen throat and deafness—anything but actual choleric symptoms—it is clearly intended to be cholera. Its origins are defined in terms reminiscent of the 1854 St. James's epidemic described by John Snow, where the epidemic started in a well that was particularly favored because the water was thought to be purer there than that from other sources: "The focus of the disease was in Petitt's well. The water, though cold, clear and sparkling, was affected by noxious gases from the drains, and had become little better than poison" (2:

137). It is traced, as was the Broad Street epidemic, to the drains of a single house. Often diseases in Victorian texts were not named out of delicacy—and denial. In turn, they tended to be defined by place rather than etiology. Yonge calls the cholera epidemic "The Water Lane Fever. People called it so as blinking its real name, but it was not the less true that it was a very pestilence in the lower part of Wilsbro'; and was prostrating its victims far and wide among gentry who had resorted to the town-hall (nearby the stricken area) within the last few weeks" (2: 132). Recognizing the role of the epidemics in nurturing professionalization, Yonge somewhat ambivalently describes a young doctor coming to a town during the epidemic as having come for the "fever pasture" (*Three Brides*, 2: 145). In other words, quite late in the century, cholera was still being used fairly unproblematically to symbolize the failure of the middle classes to nurture the health of the social sphere, which would have united the rich and poor and provided for sanitary education and improvement—even public service could be cynically used for professional advancement. Its more directly political associations, however, had largely disappeared.

Novels that used cholera as historical background include the very early *Deerbrook*, by Harriet Martineau. Smithian liberal, Malthusian, and positivist, Martineau uses cholera in her 1839 novel to symbolize the evils of superstitious, anti-scientific traditionalism. The cholera epidemic comes after the social ostracization of Dr. Hope(!) by his obtuse aristocratic patron, who resists his sanitary recommendations and disagrees with him politically (likely a source for Eliot's later and more complex portrayal of Lydgate's dilemma in *Middlemarch*), causing him to be rejected and attacked as a burker, or body snatcher, in a riot by the rural poor he is there to help. His social downfall is exacerbated by the actions of a spiteful female gossip, whose character assassination of the doctor and his family is motivated by her class snobbery. She loses her badly behaved daughter to the epidemic as a result, as she does not seek Hope's treatment for the child until too late. The cholera epidemic chastens the town, and Hope is reinstated as the proper mediator between the poor and the upper classes. Thus class snobbery, aristocratic jobbery, and the weakness of self-willed women (who are also bad mothers) are represented as social ills that cause those affected by them to pay a price in epidemic disease.

Martineau was an advocate of political economy and positivist scientific reasoning, as the novel reflects. Her other fiction for adult audiences was unabashedly didactic—a series of novelettes each devoted to illustrating a basic tenet of political economy and the principles of taxation, which were quite successful. Her only other long novel was a historical fiction about Toussaint L'Ouverture (Martineau was antislavery), and she is best known as a historian, economist, and proto-sociological journalist. Given her large historical interests, it is tempting to look for a large historical meaning in *Deerbrook*, particularly given its setting during reform and the 1832 epidemic. But the story she tells is, for the most part, a story of private life. Although Hope votes for the (winning) reform candidate over the landowner's candidate, and thus loses his practice and is persecuted by the townspeople, the force of Martineau's moral ire is directed broadly against village gossip, the evils of jealousy, superstition, and ignorance, and the mixing up of politics with social and professional life. Although Hope's family is comprised of dissenters, the Anglican minister is his broad-minded good friend, and they minister to the sick together—the Unitarian Martineau peaches religious tolerance. Religious issues enter the novel only as hysterical rumor; as Hope is charged with burking and all manner of antiestablishment evils, the landowner's wife also implies that he may be involved in church burning. No churches, however, are actually burned, and reform politics never are shown to make any difference in the novel. In fact, no specific politics are ever mentioned; the reader is simply told that Hope feels he must vote his conscience, despite his friends' caution that he should not vote, since "Nobody expects it from a medical man. Everyone knows the disadvantage to a professional man, circumstanced like you, taking any side in a party matter" (183). Martineau's negative portrayal of the Tory landowner seems to favor reform, but outside of associating it with science and her hero against the superstitious ignorance of the rural folk who are manipulated by the landowner, she cites no advantages to be had with the reform of the franchise. Cholera's powerful effect on the village is attributed to poverty and ignorance, and it serves the purpose of socially redeeming the heroic and persecuted Hope. But cholera itself is given only the implied political significance of showing up the villains for the self-serving folk they are. The only moment when the novel seems to reach toward a larger historical significance is when one of the protagonists, close to the end of both epidemic and novel, meets the town's oldest inhabitant in the churchyard. The hundred-year-old man gestures both toward the mutability of all things (he tells her of the deer and the brook, long gone, which gave the town its name) and of the persistence of life and community that will last after him. Here, then, "history" is rather the continuation of the human community rather than a specific series of significant events that change that community over time; it is a biological, rather than political view of history.

DISEASE AND THE SOCIAL BODY

In the mid-century, liberal rhetoric used disease as a sign of corruption in the social body, rot pervading the social sphere of culture and education. Discussions of politics particularly focused on questions of workers' fitness for political power. If working men were literate enough to read and judge opinions, self-controlled, able to save money and defer gratification (as demonstrated by savings accounts and insurance policies), reformers argued in the '60s, working men were fit to vote. Anti-reformers argued that many workers were ill-educated, prone to manipulation by demagogues, and too devoted to class interests. They would, by virtue of their numbers, outweigh the sober votes of the more highly cultured and therefore more politically fit elite. Novels in this period were often preoccupied with the nature of the relation between classes, and were especially attentive to the lower classes' fitness to make political judgments and take an active role in society. Elizabeth Barrett Browning's *Aurora Leigh* (1857) invokes the cholera in Aurora's first encounter with urban poverty. She goes to visit Marian, the working-class woman whom Romney, Aurora's wealthy socialist cousin, plans to marry in order to heal the breach between the classes. She is instantly recognized as an outsider in the filthy court that is Marian's home, and cursed by a woman who lives there:

> What, we pick our way
> Fine madam, with those damnable small feet!
> We cover up our face from doing good,
> As if it were our purse! . . .
> Our cholera catch you up with its cramps and spasms,
> And tumble up your good clothes, veil and all,
> And turn your whiteness dead blue. (95)

The woman's class hostility is clear, and expresses itself through the invocation of "our cholera" to strike out at the idle rich, an assault that is implicitly sexual, that "tumble[s] up" Aurora's clothes "veil and all." Disease is the weapon of the poor.

Although this scene indicates that Aurora has indeed "covered up her face," avoiding the reality of suffering and poverty, ironically, the poem ultimately justifies her attitude of slow melioration rather than Romney's attempted socialist revolution imposed from above (he founds a phalanstery in his ancestral hall and insists that the residents live by his standards of behavior, whereupon they riot and burn down his home). Real change, here, just as in Eliot's *Felix Holt* or Kingsley's *Alton Locke*, must come from change in the sphere of the social—that is, change in the domain through which the poor person understands him- or herself as a member of society, and is habituated to value cleanliness and physical self-culture. Political change of the type Romney favors is depicted as doomed to failure because it cannot change the "crooked" subjectivity of those whom it targets and therefore destines the whole society to anarchy and ruin, as befalls Leigh Hall.

Barrett Browning represents the poor as dangerous, diseased, and dirty, a "bubbling up" of subterranean sewage. When Aurora tosses money on the ground, "the whole court / Went boiling, bubbling up, from all its doors" (95).

At Romney and Marian's wedding (which fails to take place because the noble lady in love with Romney has decoyed Marian into white slavery), the poor enter the church:

> Half St. Giles in frieze
> Was bidden to meet St. James . . .
> The humours of the peccant social wound
> All pressed out, poured down upon Pimlico
> Exasperating the unaccustomed air
> With hideous interfusion. You'd suppose
> A finished generation, dead of plague,
> Swept outward from their graves into the sun,
> The moil of death upon them . . .
> They clogged the streets, they oozed into the church
> In a slow dark stream like blood . . .
> While all the aisles, alive and black with heads,
> Crawled slowly toward the altar from the street . . . Faces? . . . phew,
> We'll call them vices, festering to despairs . . .
> Twas as if you had stirred up hell
> To heave its lowest dreg-fiends uppermost
> In fiery swirls of slime,—such strangled fronts,
> Such obdurate jaws were thrown up constantly
> To twit you with your race, corrupt your blood. (123–25)

Unsurprisingly, the scene is followed by a riot, the other sign of an inadequately socialized underclass. Barrett Browning uses here the standard rhetoric—the poor are evidence of a "social wound" that festers, they are diseased and of disease, they flow like sewage, they are degenerate and "twit you with your race"—that is, show both their uncanny similarity and difference to the upper-class Britons who observe them, watching with "fear," "hate," "curiosity," "insolence," and "wondering scorn" (124). Barrett Browning has been justly criticized for the overwrought rhetoric here, but her portrayal of the upper-class watchers' casual disdain for this spectacle complicates her depiction of the poor as simply disgusting and dangerous with the accusation of the upper classes' denial of fellow feeling and responsibility for their contemporaries' plight.

Patrick Brantlinger calls Romney a cross between Dickens's horrendous philanthropists Gradgrind and Jellyby (*Spirit of Reform* 155), and there is some truth to this, although this oversimplifies the character of Romney, whose motives are far purer than either of Dickens's creations. In Romney, as Patrick Brantlinger argues, Barrett Browning rejects Fourier, Christian Socialism, organized charity, political economy, and statistics (*Spirit of Reform* 156).

Brantlinger is, however, consistently harsh in his reading—in fact, Aurora does also learn to appreciate some of the value of Romney's position as she comes to realize that the world is not so lovely a place for everyone as it has been for her. The lesson Aurora learns is to be less judgmental of others and more socially aware, as Romney must learn that he cannot create revolutions in morality by legislative fiat and that he must value the nonutilitarian achievements of art. The vision of the novel is indeed essentially conservative; the protagonist turns away from the plight of the people to cathect one person's narrative, from the problem of economic exploitation to the more sentimentally tractable one of sexual exploitation. As both Raymond Williams and Nancy Armstrong have demonstrated, this is a typical move in the social problem narrative of the period. But it also, as in Yonge, indicts the upper and middle classes for a social sin—theirs is the responsibility for educating and transforming the poor, uniting all classes in one national, social body. If Aurora's final strategy for doing this through art (from Italy, no less) is inadequate, it does not represent a complete rejection of that responsibility. Instead, she underscores the separation of the social from the realm of politics and economics and insists on the merging of Arnoldian culture—a depoliticized artistic culture—with the social. The social sphere required that people possess culture and education to appreciate it, as Ruskin insisted; the social body required physical culture and training to teach people to appreciate middle-class norms of cleanliness and comfort.

Other authors used cholera less directly, but still tied epidemic disease and especially cholera to the development of the social body and national polis. Eliot is a good example of an author who focused a good deal on the body of the individual and its relation to the health of the social body as a whole, and who used medicine and disease as persistent metaphors for bad political practice. Eliot's *Felix Holt: The Radical*, written during discussions of the second Reform Bill in the mid '60s, but set in 1832 just after the passage of reform, focuses closely on the question of politics, though it doesn't mention cholera. It is a precursor for her great novel of the early 1870s, *Middlemarch*, and rehearses many of the same themes and questions. *Middlemarch* is perhaps the most famous of all novels to mention cholera, though the actual epidemic does not feature heavily in the narrative. Instead, it is the political and social changes associated with all the events of 1832, which provide a context for the individual lives she narrates. *Middlemarch* is far longer than *Felix Holt* and is set just before and during reform.

Eliot's *Middlemarch* draws on Martineau's *Deerbrook* for many of its themes. The heroic surgeon who is persecuted for his political alliances, and whose subsequent poverty is exacerbated by marital problems, is present in both. The scenes of the women's suffering under social ostracism are also very similar. Eliot, however, makes of Lydgate less a plaster saint than Hope and dooms Rosamond to fulfill her narrow and selfish nature, whereas Martineau allows her character Hester to overcome her petty jealousy and self-absorption under the pressure of Hope's martyrdom. Whereas Martineau's tale is one of Hope's triumphant vindication, Eliot's Lydgate fails, and compromises his honor and goals. Like Martineau, Eliot is interested in questions of political economy, and frames some of the action of the novel in discussions of the responsibilities of the wealthy to the poor, though Eliot uses understated satire rather than the earnest hortatory tone more appropriate to Martineau's era and style. Eliot, like Martineau, insists on the historical setting of reform, and then avoids any specifically political conclusion, or use of the cholera to make any particular moral or scientific point about disease. However, Eliot takes Martineau's small gesture toward a long-term, evolutionary perspective and elaborates it as a fully developed, carefully theorized argument about the nature of political, social, and scientific growth in general. Whereas *Deerbrook* ultimately belies the significance of its historical setting, telling a personal story that might easily have been set in almost any period, Eliot rewrites the novel to more completely imbricate its stories of public and private life, of historical and individual idealism, failure and accommodation to historical circumstance. Eliot's two novels together are the most sustained and thoroughly theorized statement on liberal social and political questions and the body, and as such merit detailed reading here.

MEDICINE AND THE SOCIAL BODY

Literary scholar Lawrence Rothfield has read *Middlemarch* brilliantly in the light of Eliot's interest in Xavier Bichat, the French anatomist and physiologist whose work she has Lydgate, doctor and medical reformer, study. Like Bichat, Rothfield argues, Eliot's Lydgate is unable to go beyond gross tissue to the notion of the cell (which became uneasily popularized in Britain in the 1860s), although some universal "primitive tissue" is what he hopes to discover (87). He sees Eliot as using Bichat's division between organic and animal life to represent the inner and outer being, one "relatively stable," the other, caught in webs of contingency and affected by the environment, and the notion of this dual being as forming a total economy, which must either operate in an integrated way, or deteriorate (106). Lydgate fails, he suggests, because he is unable to apply his medical knowledge to his wife and his own situation. Yet, as Rothfield notes without developing the point, Lydgate also fails because scientific knowledge is not ready for the next step that Lydgate is seeking. Social and scientific evolution has not progressed to the point from which an individual might take that next step, as individuals are caught, physically, morally, and epistemologically, in the wider social web of circumstance and history.

This inability to transcend the web of historical circumstance was a theme in many of Eliot's novels, especially the later novels that tend to be set in the 1830s (or the more remote past, such as *Romola*), at moments of incipient social change. Maggie Tulliver's St. Ogg is no more ready for her largeness of sympathy than poor Dorothea's Middlemarch is ready, either for her or for reform. Felix Holt's village of Treby Magna experiences reform politics as a violent spasm of rioting and drunkenness. Like Barrett Browning, Eliot argues for developmental change, rather than change through legislative reform. Again and again, Eliot's characters must adjust their vision to the near horizon and give up their biggest dreams. When they cannot or do not, we arrive in the realm of tragedy and natural disaster, such as the flood at the end of *Mill on the Floss*. As with her characters, Eliot chides her readers for wanting too much, too soon; in *Mill*, she deprecates the importance of the lives she is narrating, only to read them as symptomatic of social evolution:

> I share with you this sense of oppressive narrowness; but it is necessary that
> we should feel it, if we care to understand how it acted . . . on young natures
> of many generations, that in the onward tendency of human things, have
> risen above the mental level of the generation before them, to which they
> have nevertheless been tied by the strongest fibres of their hearts . . . we need
> not shrink from this comparison of small things with great, for does not sci-
> ence tell us that its highest striving is after the ascertainment of a unity
> which shall bind the smallest things with the greatest? . . . there is nothing
> petty to the mind that has a large vision of relations, and to which every sin-
> gle object suggests a vast sum of conditions. (*Mill* 222–23)

Eliot instructs her audience in the reading of her work. The individual lives she narrates are not to be read separately from the larger life of the social body. Caleb Garth, the moral center of *Felix Holt*, is fascinated by the "value, the indispensable might of that myriad-headed, myriad-handed labour by which the social body is fed, clothed, and housed" (227). This is the theme of the book—the small contributions of the anonymous many, which amount to a kind of tissue growth and evolution within the organism. Dorothea, "foundress of nothing," nevertheless contributes to the growth of her society, for "the growing good of the world is partly dependent on unhistoric acts" (*Middlemarch* 766). In the crisis of her life, what saves her is her awakening to "the involuntary, palpitating life" of the larger community (721), and it is that which enables her to move beyond her own disappointed love and ambitions and lead the life of quiet contribution that is the only triumphant ending Eliot offers. Ladislaw finally becomes a political writer and strategist, working toward reform in slow increments: he becomes an "ardent public man, working well," but Eliot tempers this observation with the comment that the "young hopefulness" of reform in those days has been "much checked in our days" (*Middlemarch* 763–64). A career as the wife of a public man is a fitting end for Dorothea, whose ambition at the beginning of the novel was to be a sanitary and housing reformer avant la lettre, wanting to replace the "pig-sty cottages" on her uncle's property with "real houses fit for human beings" (*Middlemarch* 27). Felix Holt also advances a traditional liberal view of slow social melioration. Although he calls himself a radical, he is against franchise reform, believing that most men are not ready for it. He believes that "angry haste" about "evils that could only be remedied slowly, could be nothing else but obstructive" (320)—he is referring here to his own tendency to be enraged by hypocrisy, but he—and Eliot—apply the same philosophy to reform. In the "Address to Working Men, by Felix Holt," Eliot argues,

> Yes, when things are put in an extreme way, people think they know them; but, after all, they are comparatively few who see the small degrees by which these extremes are arrived at, or have the resolution and self-control to resist the little impulses by which they creep on surely toward a fatal end . . . supposing all of us to have the best intentions, we working men, as a body, run some risk of bringing evil on the nation in that unconscious manner. (appendix in *Felix Holt* 524)

Eliot, as Felix Holt, believes that workers lack the education to have developed "the treasure of refined needs" (526). Workers whose concerns are primarily bodily needs, she argues, will "debase the life of the nation," seeking those objects in preference to the greater good (526). Eliot subscribes to philosopher Herbert Spencer's notion that society develops slowly, as a single organism, by evolution. In her view, legal reforms will not make people into good citizens; the slow process of education, scientific advances, and social development will. Still, one need, like Dorothea and Ladislaw, have those ideals: "For what we call illusions are often, in truth, a wider vision of past and present realities—a willing movement of a man's soul with the larger sweep of the world's forces—a movement toward a more assured end than the chances of a single life" (*Felix Holt* 215).

Eliot's vision of society, then, is organic—society is an organism, and it has a complex relationship to the health and growth of the individual organisms who form part of its totality. Medics and naturalists have, at least potentially, a special authority to speak for and understand social development. Both Lydgate and Holt are medical men who rely on science. Lydgate is a "general practitioner" who believes in medical reform, is better educated than other provincial medics, and wants to do research and found a state-of-the-art fever hospital. He wishes to "resist the irrational severance between medical and surgical knowledge" (*Middlemarch* 132). Lydgate's desire to be part of medical reform subsides into an ordinary life with sordid compromises, partially as a result of the selfish idealism that misjudges his wife, Rosamond, seeing her merely as the creature of his own desires, and partially as a result of aligning himself with the wrong patron and showing contempt for his less scientific colleagues. Lydgate fails as a scientist, though he builds a comfortable practice, and he dies young. *Felix Holt*, like *Middlemarch*, features a medical hero (here an apothecary), who also goes against the tide of medical common sense by refusing to continue his father's business of selling a patent nostrum that Felix knows to be injurious. Where Lydgate fails, however, Holt succeeds— which is to say that he practices as an apothecary as his conscience dictates (with a sideline running a lending library for workers) and raises a son who has "a great deal more science than his father" (*Felix Holt* 507).

Felix Holt tackles reform much more directly than *Middlemarch*, using scenes typical to political novels, such as rioters whose drunkenness is due to liquor "treating" by the reform politician (reform has just been passed when the novel begins). Writing during the debates on the second Reform Bill in the '60s, Eliot returns to 1832 as the novel's setting partially in order to make a point about current issues. (This point was found to be so salient by her public that once the second bill was passed, she was asked to write an address to the newly enfranchised worker in the persona of her protagonist.) It is telling that Eliot persistently approaches the period of political reform from within the story of medical reform. Certainly, as we have seen, questions of political reform were intertwined in the public mind with questions of public health. But Eliot does not focus much on the epidemics; for her, one must use medicine to thematize reform because society itself is a body, and the nation's health or illness must be defined in terms of pathology and evolution. Politics must follow and reflect the condition of the social organism, rather than therapeutically shaping it.

Cholera, in *Middlemarch*, is only one of many indicators of societal upheaval, and is not foregrounded. Eliot's medical and scientific knowledge is precise in the novel: Rosamond's hysteria is carefully delineated, Eliot's theory of social development and of narrative realism are founded in careful study of Herbert Spencer and Bichat, and the terrain of Lydgate's scientific inquiries is painstakingly described in terms of medical theory and history, in only a few examples. Yet cholera, of all the pathologies Eliot carefully delineates, is never particularized. Instead, it is invoked in its form of public knowledge, wherein its meaning is both overdetermined and free-floating, able to attach itself to any circumstance or political conflict. Cholera arrives in town, but we do not see any cases described. Yet, the new "fever hospital" is the rock on which Lydgate's social fortunes founder, and the crisis of the novel comes at a meeting to discuss funding a cholera burial ground. At this meeting, Lydgate's patron Bulstrode is publicly challenged and disgraced.[5] It is the coming of the cholera that coincides, chapter by chapter, with Bulstrode's exposure and

Lydgate's downfall. In neither *Middlemarch* nor *Felix Holt* does the cholera ever quite arrive on stage, becoming part of the main narrative, just as reform never actually makes any difference to the actual conduct of politics. Yet, in both novels, disease of the individual and social body is thematically connected throughout the work. As Rothfield says, Eliot's tale of Lydgate is a "pathologically organic plot," which "takes the shape of a descending arc in which the individual is progressively disarticulated" (108–09), and to some extent, this is also the story of society's young hope for reform. Still, there is Ladislaw, the other outsider in the novel, who makes better choices, and like Dorothea, reaches outward toward the wider life of the social body rather than inward: "political writing, political speaking, would get a higher value now public life was going to be wider and more national" (*Middlemarch* 463).

In *Middlemarch*, reform is also associated with no particular idea in the minds of voters (or in the mind of Brooke, the reform candidate), and is compromised by association with the most foolish and fiscally selfish, though good-natured, character, who himself holds several contradictory views at any given time. One tenant, excited by alcohol and political talk, threatens to attack Brooke, and this working-class violence is the only visible impact of reform itself, as it is in *Felix Holt*, in which newly enfranchised and drunken voters riot. Political rhetoric is likened to a drug or alcohol itself—potent to cure or sicken. It is "muddy political talk, dangerously disturbing," which the belligerent tenant takes with too much alcohol on market day (*Middlemarch* 359). Lydgate and Ladislaw argue about reform, Lydgate arguing that reform is not scientific medicine, but "hocus pocus," and that "society can't be cured" by it (424). Ladislaw successfully argues against Lydgate's position by comparing political reform to medical reform, and adjacent chapters 45 and 46 are about Lydgate's attempted medical reforms and the Reform Bill itself, respectively.[6]

By connecting her idealistic protagonists to reform—Dorothea to cottage reform, Ladislaw to political reform, and Lydgate to medical reform—Eliot connects the body and sanitation to the social body. By constraining them all to accept incremental rather than sweeping change, however, she insists on the primacy of slow, evolutionary melioration over revolution, scientific or otherwise. Science, like other new knowledge, is valuable in the hands of experts. In the mouths of the general public, such discourse becomes at best, despoiled of meaning, and at worst, dangerous. As the tide of public feeling turns against Lydgate, and people begin to accuse him of possibly being a "burker" of bodies, Eliot makes a telling comparison to mid-century sanitary rhetoric, stepping deliberately out of the time frame of the narrative in an aside:

> some of the particulars [reported about Lydgate were] . . . of that impressive order of which the significance is entirely hidden, like a statistical amount without the standard of comparison, but with a note of exclamation on the

end. The cubic feet of oxygen swallowed yearly by a full-grown man—what a shudder they might have created in Middlemarch circles! "Oxygen! Nobody knows what that may be—is it any wonder the cholera has got to Dantzic? And yet there are people who say quarantine is no good!" (*Middlemarch* 403)

The preoccupation with how much air one body used was the preoccupation of a much later time—here, in a rare explicit comparison, Eliot denounces the popular misunderstanding of science in her own time through her ridicule of the benighted provincials of nearly four decades earlier. Lydgate is also rumored (correctly) to dispense no drugs, thus simultaneously offending by setting himself at the level of a physician (instead of a surgeon-apothecary), and offending his brethren the surgeon-apothecaries by implying the critique of their practice (as they make their fees principally on the drugs they dispense and not on their advice or attendance). Finally, of course, he offends many of his clients who feel that they are getting less matter for their money and being forced to pay for what would be free elsewhere—medical advice.

Eliot is most interested in narrating private lives, but "there is no private life which has not been determined by a wider public life" (*Felix Holt* 75). In these novels, reform often seems to exist merely as a backdrop for private stories. However, it is important to realize that this influence on which Eliot insists flows in both directions—it is private lives, often forgotten ones like Dorothea's, that make up "the largeness of the world and the manifold wakings of men to labour and endurance" (*Middlemarch* 722). Her persistent return to 1832, and her desire to write, in *Felix Holt*, a novel about reform and politics, belies any narrow emphasis of individual psychology over larger issues in her novels. Indeed, her novels, especially her later ones, were all focused on the large issues of evolution and the relation of individual development to the larger social and historical milieu. But it was not through politics that she thought national improvement would take place, but through the development of individuals, laboring together for the good of the social body. Like Ruskin, Arnold, and the sanitary reformers of mid-century, she believed that national improvement must emerge out of the development of "refined needs," and the management of desire. Desire was a principal theme for Eliot, and she turned a clinical eye on its vagaries. Misplaced desire, for Eliot, leads to every abuse of nature from bad marriages to drug and alcohol abuse, and misplaced political desire leads to violence.

DESIRE AND ADDICTION

As Eliot says in *Mill on the Floss*, "Good society, floated on gossamer wings of light irony, is of very expensive production, requiring nothing less than a wide and arduous national life condensed in unfragrant deafening factories. . . . This wide national life is based entirely on emphasis—the emphasis of want, which urges it into all the activities necessary for the maintenance of good society and light irony." This "want,"—basic material desires and needs operating well below the "refined needs" recommended to the working man as the basis for fit use of the franchise—when frustrated of its legitimate fulfillment, leads to the need for "an emphatic belief. . . . Some have an emphatic belief in alcohol and seek their *ekstasis* or standing ground in gin." Bad politics, opium, alcohol, and gambling are the outlets to which characters turn in Eliot's novels. Lydgate, under the pressure of his miserable marriage, tries opium, and under the pressure of his financial needs, tries gambling. Gwendolyn Harleth gambles out of craving for excitement (in *Daniel Deronda*), and as many critics have shown, an astonishing number of Eliot's characters abuse alcohol. Kathleen McCormack has traced Eliot's fascination with opium addiction, and the use of inappropriate drugs as a metaphor for inappropriate politics, especially in *Felix Holt*. Sexual desire, when inappropriate, is likened to disease in *Middlemarch*, and indeed the progress of Lydgate and Rosamond's courtship depends on Fred's typhoid (often thought to presage a cholera epidemic, and, in fact, the cholera epidemic arrives soon after). The loss of Lydgate's ambition in consequence is described as infection as well: "Nothing in the world more subtle than the process of their gradual change! In the beginning they inhaled it unknowingly; you and I may have sent some of our breath toward infecting them . . . or perhaps it came with the vibrations from a woman's glance" (*Middlemarch* 131).

Desire is the great theme of Eliot's work, and she sees desire as the motive force of all human action. "We are all of us imaginative in one form or another, for images are the brood of desire" (293), Eliot reminds her readers in *Middlemarch*. In *Felix Holt*, desire gone astray destroys, as Eliot uses a sensation plot about a woman with a secret adulterous past—in this case, the politician Harold Transome's mother. Materially well off, but comfortless and powerless over her own fate, Mrs. Transome's addiction is to power, as Eliot makes clear: "what could then sweeten the days to a hungry, much exacting self like Mrs. Transome's? Under protracted ill every living creature will find something that makes a comparative ease, and even when life seems woven of pain, will convert the fainter pang into a desire. Mrs. Transome . . . found the opiate for her discontent in the exertion of her will about smaller things" (30). Throughout the novel, Eliot emphasizes that it is not just substances that are addictive, but desire itself.

Early in her married life, Mrs. Transome had an affair with her lawyer. Mrs. Transome's appetite for the lawyer, Jermyn, stems not only from frustration with her husband, but from frustrated maternal desire. Indeed, when Jermyn's son Harold is born, she desires the death of her licit but cretinous firstborn, so that Harold may inherit the wealth and name to which he bears no biological right. But the first son's idiocy itself is spawned out of inappropriate sexual desire on the part of a male Transome. Foreshadowing the 1890s' indictment of syphilitic fathers, Eliot makes clear in her introductory chapter that the Transome degeneration is due to "some quickly satiated desire that survives, with the life in death of old paralytic vice, to see itself cursed by its woeful progeny" (10). This degeneration can also be seen in old Tommy Trounsem, the alcoholic last living Transome of his line.

Scorning conventional morality as "stupid and drug-like," fit only for the social control of inferiors, Mrs. Transome has no moral defenses against her own desires, which cannot be satisfied. Mrs. Transome, who is constantly described as "hungry" with "a void which could not be filled," had hoped her son would fill that void and "give unity to her life . . . but the mother's early raptures had lasted but a short time, and even while they lasted there had grown up in the midst of them a hungry desire, like a black poisonous plant feeding in the sunlight,—the desire that her first . . . child should die. . . . Such desires make life a hideous lottery, where every day may turn up a blank" (23). Mrs. Transome's affair with Jermyn and even maternity of Harold take the place of opiates or gambling; they pretend to sate but actually create new desire. The focus on desire as a danger leading to pathological conditions of the body such as addiction hearkens back to the earlier rhetoric of sin, in which intemperance was the predisposing cause of individual susceptibility to epidemic disease. Here, temperance takes a new and more encompassing form, but still focuses on inappropriate desires, and still connects the morality of self-control to preservation from disease.

However, the avoidance of appetite is not Eliot's answer either. After an initial period of debauchery, Felix attempts to avoid even socially sanctioned desire; "he evaded calamity by choosing privation" (356), preferring to live on turnips rather than be tempted by sexual desire into marriage, which he believes must inevitably compromise his principles by forcing him to meet the needs of a wife and children. Felix's radicalism initially appears to be assisted by this principled rejection of social investments that imply social constraints. As Jermyn muses, he is "a young man with so little of the ordinary Christian motives as to making an appearance and getting on in the world, that he presented no handle to any judicious and respectable person who might be willing to make use of him" (185). He is willing to live frugally to the point of asceticism.

Felix must be brought by the end of the novel to acknowledge his desire for Esther and renounce his earlier renunciation of domesticity and paternity. Temperance and self-control are achieved, not through the avoidance of temptation and desire, but through daily struggle and compromise. As is usual with Eliot, the principal problems of desire are situated in the woman poised on the brink of adulthood. Through Esther, as she will later do with Dorothea Brooke, Maggie Tulliver, and Gwendolen Harleth, Eliot points out clearly that the same desire that leads to spiritual growth leads to addiction; the goal is to channel it properly. Like Dorothea's desire to contribute to the world, which initially leads her to offer herself on Casaubon's unworthy altar but finally brings her into the safe, if small, harbor of Ladislaw's political career, Esther's "hunger" for higher things, initially and harmfully focused on material objects, later becomes focused on spiritual development and Felix. Her hunger, therefore is both the basis of both her goodness and her temptation: "it comes in so many forms in this life of ours—the knowledge that there is something sweetest and noblest of which we despair, and the sense of something present that solicits us with an immediate and easy indulgence" (*Felix Holt* 406): in this case, Harold Transome's courtship. When she tells him playfully that she only likes what she cannot have, he offers her a superficially respectable temperance in answer: "I am very fond of things that I can get. And I never longed much for anything out of my reach. . . . Some are given to discontent and longing, others to securing and enjoying. And let me tell you, the discontented longing style is unpleasant to live with" (410). Offering her the drug of an easy material well-being, he requires that she give up that hunger that makes her, for Eliot, most fully human.

Hitherto, Eliot suggests, this natural desire for "higher things" has been a force that popular-Benthamite social engineers have attempted to manage, without respect for the humanity and multifarious desires of individuals, and therefore without success: "Fancy what a game chess would be if all the chessmen had passions and intellects, more or less small and cunning. . . . You might be the longest headed of deductive reasoners, and yet you might be beaten by your own pawns . . . especially . . . if you depended arrogantly on your mathematical imagination, and regarded your passionate pieces with contempt" (*Felix Holt* 278). The point for Eliot, (as it was of course for Bentham himself), is to acknowledge desire and harness it to social ends. These ends are not mere material wealth or political power (as Felix says of the vote, "Not yet! Something else before all that"), but an Arnoldian vision of culture that transmutes appetite into an evolutionary force in the service of humanity. Without that culture, desires beyond the basic needs of food and drink tend to become vices: "the multiplying brood begotten by parents who have been left without all teaching save that of a too-craving body, without all well-being save the fading delusions of drugged beer and gin" (*Felix Holt* 492). Eliot recommends culture as the substitute for drugs, urging her audience to foster and preserve "the treasure of refined needs" (495). Looking beyond the sanitary question per se (though she nods to it in making Dorothea a cottage reformer), Eliot focuses on the mid-century question of bringing the lower classes to have the same desires and tastes as their social superiors. Once the immediate threat of filth was brought under control, it was the habits and appetites of the poor that were believed to require moderation, so that they might eventually be incorporated into the larger community without threat. Addiction is used by Eliot—and, as we shall see, by other authors as well—to trope the misdirection of desire toward meeting "low" appetites rather than directing it toward ennobling ambition. Addiction and disease both are used to represent the physical causes and effects of the selfishness and small-mindedness that weakens community.

Throughout the period, novelists that advanced a sanitarian agenda tended to use national rhetoric more, invoking cleanliness as a sign of the enlightened civilization of Britain. The rhetoric of nation was stronger in these works and through the '50s than in Martineau, Eliot, or Yonge, who are more interested in a broad sense of community that is not explicitly defined as nation. Although Eliot's persistent return to the themes and era of reform, paired with a medical hero (who is, in one case, also a political radical), suggests the novels positioned themselves as national history, nation itself is not invoked as a project. It is the "social body" that Eliot specifically names, in part as a nod to the historical preoccupation of the 1830s with political economy, but more importantly, as a theme of the novels themselves. It is the development of a social body and the relation of the individual to it that interests Eliot, and the relationship of that body to national identity, or to politics, is secondary for her. In *Middlemarch*, this is manifested in the development of characters like Dorothea, and in *Felix Holt*, it is much more explicitly linked to the question of the franchise. But in both, the body and its health as a metaphor for the community and its social well-being are fundamental concerns. Because the political health of the community is based on social health and not on legislation or enfranchisement, the social relations of the classes and the moral health of individuals becomes a more compelling way to talk about politics than discussion of political change itself. Eliot uses medical science as a stand-in for political health in part because she sees the social body as an organism, best described in clinical terms. But it works so well and seems so natural in part because the question of health had become basic to that of the Condition of England. The medic and the politician were both at best "public men," contributing to the well-being and guidance of the social body.

8

Kingsley

Nation, Gender, and the Body

THE HEALTHY MASCULINE ENGLISH BODY became the foundation and index of the healthy nation in the nineteenth-century novel. Scholars such as Lenore Davidoff and Catherine Hall, James Eli Adams, and John Tosh have characterized the mid-century as a time of crisis in masculine self-definition among the middling classes. These writers have stressed the roles of self-control, sexual continence, and domesticity in defining the manly (or gentlemanly) man. Gendered domesticity was key to national identity in this period; although the love of man for his patria was to be based in the steadying influence of home and family, the woman who metonymically stood for these values was passive, supposedly neither an agent of nation nor of empire. As McClintock complains, "All too often in male nationalisms, gender differences between women and men serve to symbolically define the limits of national difference and power between men. . . . Excluded from direct influence as national citizens, women are subsumed into the national body politic as its boundary and metaphoric limit" (354). I am less concerned here with nationalism per se than with discourses of national identity (on which, of course, nationalisms depend), for which McClintock's observations are equally pertinent. Concerns about gender and domesticity were particularly clear in novelistic discourse about the nation and its health. In this chapter, I give special attention to a particular example and influential producer of such discursive formations: Charles Kingsley and his insistently masculine, heterosexual "Muscular Christianity."

Charles Kingsley (1819–1875), Broad Church Anglican minister, sometime Chartist radical, sanitarian, naturalist, historian, and novelist, was at the heart of the sanitary movement, representing two of its most powerful components—that of the natural scientist and that of the minister. He is also, however, important for his work in the related areas of poor relief and workers' rights, and, perhaps most crucially, as the most powerful spokesperson for the philosophies of "Muscular Christianity"—a term he at first disliked, but which gained so much popularity he later learned to accept it. Muscular Christianity and related ideas both expressed and strongly shaped understandings of gender and nation in the mid-nineteenth century, and continued to be crucial to imperial masculinity through the turn of the twentieth. Kingsley's novels, widely influential in their own time, provide an excellent example of the elaboration of these rhetorics in that privileged mirror of bourgeois subjectivity, the three-volume novel.

Bruce Haley shows how the *mens sana in corpore sano* became a doctrine of holistic moral and physical health in the Victorian period. He also shows how healthfulness comes to be gendered masculine in this period, just as illness is often gendered feminine: "*mens sana* means manliness or pluck, a quality similar to physical strength or courage and dependent on them. . . . 'To be a nation of good animals,' Herbert Spencer wrote, 'is the first condition to national prosperity'" (Haley 22). Mind and body were inseparable in this period in terms of health and disease etiology—mental stress could lead to fever, physical uncleanliness would lead to moral turpitude. Samuel Smiles, another proponent of exercise for manliness and success and author of the wildly popular book *Self-Help: With Illustrations of Character and Good Conduct* (1859), also claimed health as a national trait (Haley 207). As Haley points out, "Because robustness was a national [English] and therefore classless trait, it was the natural sign of the true gentleman, not only a virtue but an emblem of virtue" (207). The reverse, of course, was also true—the unhealthy, spindly, dirty worker was neither virtuous nor, quite, English.

Charles Kingsley, like many other Victorians, insisted that proper, socialized masculinity emerged out of the rigid control of animal instinct. Unlike some other writers, however, he repudiated the idealization of a monkish abstinence in favor of a regulatory but fully embraced domestic heterosexuality. It was important, if masculine self-control was to be worth anything, that those animal instincts be extremely powerful. Thus, the civilized man depended for his identity on the notion that he was potentially, and at any moment, a savage. If a man is unable to control such impulses, he is feminized by the very source of his masculinity, as someone ruled by impulse and emotion. The man who became so civilized that he no longer had such bestial instincts, however, was also feminized for lack of any need to restrain himself. No wonder the boundary line between beast and man, savage and civilized gentleman required such careful scrutiny! Kingsley's lesser characters learn this self-control through homosocial relations, (hero worship and so forth);

his heroes, however, as males without clear peers, instinctively have a great deal of honorable masculine self-control, but must learn to focus this splendid energy through love of a woman. Kingsley's notion of woman is somewhat Goethean—the eternal feminine lures to perfection—and for Kingsley, this means heroic action to win her sexual affections in marriage. The heroic man is physically healthy, which also almost automatically means he is morally upright, for as Kingsley often asserted, "your soul makes your body." The man who is perfectly healthy does what is right by instinct, and then requires only the love of a good woman to awaken in him the higher spirituality that can be achieved only through altruistic dedication to a higher purpose. Finally, through suffering, the hero learns the limits of his own (considerable) powers, and this wins him to an understanding and acceptance of God's guidance, as God is the ultimate alpha male.

Although its insistence on the healthiness of male sexuality and the naturalness of the religious instinct for right action were somewhat different from other existing, more ascetic theories of manliness, Kingsley's representation of woman as muse and enabler, and not much else, and of the need for homosocial bonding and hero worship is quite Carlylean. In any case, regardless of the widespread tendency to poke fun at Kingsley's Muscular Christians, the Charles Kingsley/Thomas Hughes-style hero—unreflective, physically strong, and loving exertion for its own sake, instinctively honorable and obsessively clean—was recognized as a specifically British type, and most particularly, an English type. The overgrown schoolboy who was to become the ideal of the imperial hero, the quintessential John Bull, was epitomized by Kingsley's heroes, who managed to combine that which was considered manly with Christian morality without leaching all of the appeal out of the characters. In short, Kingsley's work crystallized something important about Britons' sense of what British men were and, perhaps, should be. Kingsley believed in the concept that a healthy (male) animal was more likely to develop proper Christian feelings, and that the truest religion was based in intuitive right reactions grounded in a healthy organism rather than intellectual consideration and choice.

Kingsley early became interested in the problems of the poor and flirted with Chartism and Christian Socialism, which aimed at reclaiming religion "for the people" and as an inherently political institution (Brantlinger, *Spirit of Reform* 132). As Brantlinger points out, Kingsley makes this connection in 1850 in *Alton Locke* (133). Brantlinger ridicules Kingsley's Chartist sympathies (*Spirit of Reform*, 139), and with good reason—ultimately, the Church of England, of which Kingsley was a minister, was an anti-Chartist institution. However, Kingsley's position was hardly unusual. Like many middle-class liberals and radicals, he combined for a while belief in radical change in legislative privileges with an unshaken faith in the rightness of the existing social order. Sooner or later, progress would correct what he saw as problems incidental to the structure of society, which were consequent on mistaken notions of natural law. Many readers have found him intellectually confused; yet, his position was absolutely typical of a number of activists who considered themselves Christians, but who also embraced liberal politics and a faith in scientific progress. His predilection for specific and pragmatic solutions within existing institutions and respect for natural, scientific laws, as well as his long-standing commitment to the well-being of the poor, made sanitary reform a natural interest for such an avid naturalist. It also contributed to his embrace of racial and degeneration theories.

NATION AND THE SOCIAL BODY

Donald Hall notes the importance of the social body metaphor in Kingsley's Chartist novel, *Alton Locke*, where it is used to subordinate and control working-class political dissidence (51); this metaphor remained crucial for Kingsley throughout his work. It is worth paying some attention to the principal elaborator of this metaphor in the mid-century—philosopher Herbert Spencer. Spencer was at odds with Kingsley in many ways—Kingsley could not stomach Spencer's rigid free-market survival-of-the-fittest position, and Spencer derided the hero worship so dear to Carlyle and his followers as a barbaric emotion befitting an oppressive society (see *Social Statics* 376–78). But the penetration of Kingsley's prose by a multitude of Spencerian ideas and images suggests a substantial influence, even if some of it may have come through Spencer's popularizers rather than directly. Spencer's fascination for the latest in medical, histological, and evolutionary science pervaded his work (as it did his close friend George Eliot's writing), and *Social Statics*, first published in 1850, proved vastly influential. In addition to the already fairly popular formulation that there was a "homogeneity of national character. . . . In whichever rank you see corruption, be assured it equally pervades all ranks— be assured it is the symptom of a bad social diathesis. While the virus of depravity exists in one part of the body politic, no other part can remain healthy" (208), he argued that laws and social structures were molded by a state's "character" and that, as the highest form of society was a democracy, attempts at reform, Chartism, and abolition reflected the evolution of a "moral sense" (215–16).

For Spencer, the highest state of society required the most advanced condition of "individuation" of each person, which in turn required the greatest "mutual dependence" (397). He compares the despotism of the czar to that of American slave owners, who are in turn "shackled" by the requirements of coercion (398)—"The tyrant is nothing but a slave turned inside out" (92). (Certainly, many of these ideas and comparisons were circulating widely in

British writing; still, the organization of examples in Kingsley's 1857 novel, *Two Years Ago*, evinces a strong similarity to Spencer's earlier work.) Finally, Spencer argues that the social body, like the individual body, is made up of "innumerable microscopic organisms, which possess a kind of independent vitality, which grow by imbibing nutriment from the circulating fluids, and which multiply . . . by spontaneous fission. The whole process of development . . . is fundamentally a perpetual increase in the number of these cells . . . that gradual decay witnessed in old age is in essence a cessation of this increase" (403). Here again, then, the influence of Bichatian tissue theory is evident. This is even more strongly reflected in Spencer's frequently repeated argument that "Nature demands that every being be self-sufficing. All that are not so, nature is perpetually withdrawing by death" (339). Although Kingsley waged tireless war in the mid-century on political economists who adopted some version of this view, he evidences this same—if Christianized—emphasis on self-sufficiency in *Two Years Ago* (1857). In 1852, Spencer writes,

> the process of modification has effected, and is effecting, decided changes in all organisms subject to modifying influences . . . any existing species—animal or vegetable—when placed under conditions different from its previous ones, *immediately begins to undergo certain changes fitting it for the new conditions* . . . in successive generations these changes continue; until, ultimately, the new conditions become the natural ones. (his emphasis, Essay, *Leader*)

Certainly this generally Lamarckian evolution is that which Kingsley embraces.

By the end of the '50s, Kingsley would be much closer to Spencer's hard-nosed doctrines than he was at the beginning, though he never accepted Spencer's Social Darwinism. The ideas that emerged in Kingsley from these and related intellectual sources are four: a Lamarckian vision of acquired characteristics; a modified Bichatian understanding of life as a process in which tissue was generated to match these acquired characteristics and maladaptive "scar" tissue died and must be sloughed; the linkage between these processes in an individual and social body, from which the individual took its meaning and to which, in order to be healthy, it must remain in right relation; and the crucial identification between an integrated social body and nation. To this, he adds the Carlylean/Mauricean concerns about the role of masculinity in nation building that anchor his oeuvre, a series of novels devoted to mythologizing the origins of English Protestant nationhood.

Kingsley was obsessively interested in the nature of nation and the elements that constituted national progress. This fascination was elaborated in part in terms of foundational narratives that were then marked out in terms of racial theory and ethnic history, much as they were for Carlyle and other mid-Victorian thinkers. As historian Mark Harrison notes, Victorian theories of race are difficult to pin down, but the largely climatic determinism of the late eighteenth and early nineteenth century "was reformulated in less flexible and [more] hereditarian terms" (*Climates* 120), and in new theories advancing multiple, racially distinct origins from humanity. Harrison argues that

> Racial theory . . . tended to encourage a certain fatalism among Europeans; a fatalism which sat uneasily with the more interventionist visions of empire which emerged in the 1820s and 30s, on the back of evangelical Christianity and reformist liberalism. Racial theories rested on the belief that human characteristics were essentially unvarying, whereas reformers tended to think of them as capable of improvement. (*Climates* 220)

The wavering, though increasing, commitment to a biologically essential conception of race that many Victorian thinkers displayed had to be reconciled with a broadly catholic view of Christianity for Kingsley, which he finally resolved with a combination of appeals to a racialist and Protestant vision of English origins with a kind of evolutionary monism that, in 1857, used race as a de-essentialized, mutable developmental marker.

Nation then, resolved itself into a social body that defined itself developmentally in relation to a particular task. Various sins of selfishness and dependence caused stagnation or degeneration, both nationally and individually, and sanitary problems were one of the symptoms of such deficiency. Kingsley's vision of nation hooked the two missions, social and imperial, together in a rhetoric that negotiated between the 1832 rhetoric of the Anglican church and the radicals and the 1850s rhetoric of the sanitarians. He used the metaphor of the suffering body to emblematize the task of the nation: to heal itself, "making" a better body through spiritual and material development.

TWO YEARS AGO: NATION AND MASCULINITY

Two Years Ago was one of Kingsley's more popular novels. The action is largely set in the time leading up to the onset of both the third cholera epidemic and the Crimean War in 1855, two years before the publication of the novel. Ostensibly, the novel is principally about surgeon Tom Thurnall, a Kingsleyan muscular hero who fights cholera with science and, after a lifetime of careless daredevil heroics, finds God when his sense of self-reliance is broken during the war. The cholera and the war, as is typical in religious novels and tracts, turn out to be blessings as the trials by which male characters find both fortitude and faith.

However, this more-or-less typical story is embedded within the framing story of another issue, in which Kingsley in fact invests more narrative energy:

U.S. slavery, which not only provides the basis of one of the novel's several principal plots, but becomes the underlying metaphor for the principal theme of struggle for national and personal evolution. Critics have rarely commented much on the racial politics of the novel, and when they have, they have tended simply to note its inclusion in the genre of British abolitionist literature, and its typical Victorian fascination with the figure of the beautiful, sexually exploited octoroon.[1] The abolition storyline has often been seen (even by its author) as completely eccentric to the main plotlines of the book. But the abolitionist narrative is more than simply a single, wayward strand of this ambitiously complex novel; it is the frame of the entire work, and slavery is the dominant metaphor throughout the novel for the irrationality and brutality at the heart of modernity that taints it and must be expunged for spiritual growth to take place and national destiny to be fulfilled.

Slavery, and its analogues in the novel—hysteria, addiction, disease—emasculates, barbarizes, and derationalizes, undermining the project of national progress through social improvement—sanitary reform, education, colonization—that Kingsley identifies as the central project of both Britain and her "child," the United States. Slavery, like addiction or disease, implies the vulnerability of the self to the abject, whether as dependence on a drug, economic dependence on the degrading practice of slavery, or invasion by the unnatural "disorder" of disease. The novel invokes sanitary and abolition rhetoric in the name of national development and couches the story of national development in terms of individual masculinity and spiritual/physical regeneration. Once again, the presence of cholera indexes dysfunction in the relation between classes, and poor government, whether of the community or the self.

Masculinity in *Two Years Ago* is developed by the struggle for national purification and identity, just as the mark of national weakness is the feminization of the men and the need for women to step out of their place into the male role of public speaker, as the African American Marie does when she is whipped for speaking out as a slave, "speaking as a woman should speak" (91)—probably, against sexual exploitation—and again by going on stage to advance the cause of abolition.

Two key male characters, presented as admirable in their ways, each bear an emasculating weakness. Stangrave, who courts Marie without knowing at first that she is octoroon, is an accomplished and wealthy American who has not wanted the fuss and bother of opposing slavery directly, even though he knows it is a moral blot on his nation. Frank Headley, the Anglican curate, is a slight, elegant, consumptive but well-intentioned man who despairs of gaining any orthodox command over the hard-bitten dissenting fishermen of Aberalva. Frank's flaw is the narrowness of his Anglicanism, but the narrator warns the reader to honor his ideal "of a perfect polity, a 'Divine and wonderful Order,' linking earth to heaven, and to the very throne of him who died for men; witnessing to each of its citizens what the world tries to make him forget, namely, that he is the child of God himself" (*Two Years Ago* 85). Here is a Christianized vision of Spencer's perfectly developed society, a "perfect polity" in which each is a "citizen." The narrator explains that if the principal protagonist Tom Thurnall—who also honors order above all—is one "pole of the English character," Frank is the other, "as good an Englishman as" Tom and with much to teach him.

If Frank is the good man who, because of physical shortcomings, must be physically masculinized, Arthur to Tom Thurnall's Tom Brown, John Briggs (later called Elsley Vavasour), serves as the unsalvageable feminized man, and is opposed to hero Tom Thurnall from the start. Tom is the typical Kingsley hero, quintessentially English and athletic, and John is physically beautiful but vain, nervous, and artistic rather than sports oriented—a bit of a dandy: full of "nasty, effeminate, un-English foppery!" (16), as one character opines. Both start off as medics, but John leaves this career path early on. John's wool-gathering intellect manifests itself in carelessness with prescriptions; when, as an adolescent apprentice to an apothecary, he gives the local banker a black draught instead of his cough medicine, the banker hyperbolically accuses him of having given him cholera. This disorderliness, and inattention to detail, along with masculine selfishness, is indeed what causes cholera later in the novel.

John/Elsley eventually becomes a poet, and the especial target of Kingsley's wrath. Early on, he shows promise by writing about London's poor (rather like Alton Locke), but with success, he withdraws his attention from them and writes of "sufferers of a more poetic class"—Italy under the yoke of Austria, to be specific—and changes his name to Elsley Vavasour. But with no practical ability or understanding of politics, Elsley finds little worth saying. Because he is out of touch with the world around him, he is shocked and terrified when Tom mentions that cholera is coming and that he reckons on increased income in the event: "'Good Heavens . . . you do not talk of that frightful scourge—so disgusting, too, in its character—as a matter of profit and loss? It is sordid, cold-hearted!'" (*Two Years Ago* 161). Elsley is most horrified by the character of the disease, showing once again his inability to face painful realities, and therefore, to impose order on disorder. Elsley's weakness finally expresses itself in an unjustified jealousy of his wife, which causes him to run off and become an opium addict, mirroring the many minor characters in this novel who demonstrate their inadequate British self-control through addiction to opiates and alcohol.

Elsley's inferiority to "real men" is attributable to the decadent effects of an exhausted European hyper-culturalism expressed in his interest in spasmodic poetry and unmanly shame over his class origins. Elsley has no interest in nature, no ability to see its beauties, nor does he cultivate his own body:

he lacks all key attributes of the Kingsleyan Muscular Christian. When Tom advises Elsley to exercise, and is answered petulantly in reply, he thinks, "'You touchy ass. . . . If we were in the blessed state of nature right now, wouldn't I give you ten minutes double thonging, and then set you to work, as the runaway nigger did his master'" (*Two Years Ago* 196). Vitality is in the working fishermen of Aberalva and in Tom as worker; in a "state of nature" he would dominate and enslave the effeminate Elsley, as, perhaps, in a state of nature, American slaves would dominate their masters, who have become effeminate through dependence on their service—again, a kind of addiction. The novel persistently locates authentic masculinity in the body of the worker, the professional, and the soldier, as opposed to the aristocrat or aesthete. As C. J. W. L. Wee points out, this recourse to the body of the "savage" or "primitive," as Kingsley thought of Africans, as superior to the decadent European, is a common device of Kingsley's, who is then challenged to meld his romantic longing for a primitive manly vigor with his mid-century liberal privileging of the cultured European ideal.

But if Elsley's response to the advent of cholera is inappropriate, so is Tom's matter-of-fact humorousness. Following Kingsley's earlier Crimean War allegory set in Elizabethan England, which sent the English "Westward Ho" to extend their empire and free the natives from the evil Spanish "enslavers," this novel sends its heroes "Eastward Ho," as it notes several times, on basically the same errand (the enslavers being, this time, Russian). Published just before the Sepoy Mutiny, the novel designates Eastern service and the command of "black" troops in India as that which makes a man.[2] Major Campbell, one of the mentor figures of the novel, achieves his manliness through this trajectory. (Although Tom has been Eastward, he has gone as a mercenary and not in the service of a larger cause; he therefore remains essentially boyish and morally undeveloped.) The major exemplifies the appropriate response to cholera—he is horrified, but not frightened, by the prospect of cholera: "It is too dreadful! I have seen it in India—among my own men—among the natives. Good heavens! I never shall forget—and to meet the fiend again here, of all places of the world! I fancied it so clean, and healthy, swept by fresh sea breezes'" (*Two Years Ago* 269). He immediately asks what can be done to prevent it, but also exhorts Tom to "think of God!" (269). Like Tom, the major has experience of the disease and does not fear it, but unlike Tom, it has not caused him to adopt a blasé or cynical attitude.

That Aberalva is headed for sanitary trouble is evident from the first chapters of the novel, when the narrator describes the local children playing in the quay pool into which the sewer serving, as the narrator emphasizes, "1500 souls," empties its unfragrant contents (37). The state of the streets and what it portends is immediately compared to the condition of the British soldiers then steaming toward Russia: an unknowing movement toward military and epidemic disaster. Aberalva is also filled with addicts, all of whom suffer rather horribly from cholera. Squire Trebooze is as pickled as his name suggests, and is "saved" from killing himself with alcohol poisoning by his disabling delirium tremens. Luckily, he finds salvation in the military. The local apothecary, Mr. Heale, and his wife, a drunkard and laudanum addict respectively, have less good fortune, dying in the epidemic. The presence of addicts in the novel suggest a state of illness, nonindependence in the individual. Even Marie, the octoroon heroine, demands a vacation, emphasizing that with her "craving for exhilaration, the capability of self-indulgence, in our wild Tropic blood" she needs rest, for she fears she is beginning "to want stimulants" to keep up her strength under the strain of acting (*Two Years Ago* 207). Here, however, unlike in novels of the late '40s and early '50s, substance dependence does not signify social protest, but the personal irresponsibility that creates an inadequate society and weakens nation. In short, he is moving toward the 1860s liberalism of Arnold and Eliot, a politics of personal transformation. In Kingsley (as in Eliot), addiction represents an unconscionable self-absorption, an attempt to fulfill desire without appeal to a higher aspiration toward God or community. It is an expression of the same kind of self-centeredness that results in the refusal to make sanitary reforms, a trusting to the self's ability to overcome threats to the social body.

"Were you ever condemned to spin ropes of sand to all eternity . . . or to extract the cube roots of a million or two of hopeless surds, . . . or last, and worst of all, to work the Nuisances Removal Act? Then you can enter, as a man and a brother, into the sorrows of Tom Thurnall" (*Two Years Ago* 222). Tom finds the act impossible to enforce, as a matter that "touches the pocket" of the pillars of the community. The old doctor does not want to offend his customers and affirms that it is the judgment of God, as does the local Evangelical preacher, who is planning to found a profitable revival on the epidemic. Frank the curate "already believed his [Tom's] doctrines, as an educated London parson of course would" but has little influence (226), and merely gives his enemies ammunition: "the Brianite preacher denounced him . . . as a German Rationalist, who impiously pretended to explain away the Lord's visitation . . . his rival, of another denomination, who was a fanatic on the teetotal question, denounced him as bitterly for supporting the cause of drunkenness, by attributing cholera to want of cleanliness, while all rational people knew its true source was intemperance" (*Two Years Ago* 228). A "man and a brother," Tom is "enslaved" by the selfishness of community members, each of whom wishes either not to lose money or actively to make a profit on the epidemic. He struggles for a sanitary abolition of slavery to disease, as sanitation is figured as the expulsion of a barbaric enslavement to the body's wastes.

As a medic (he is a surgeon, but is often referred to simply as a doctor by himself and the other characters), Tom represents scientific reason and order imposed upon the social domain. Tom explains his vocation to Frank in terms that clearly take as his territory one far beyond "disease" as we would think of it today:

> it's a sort of sporting with your true doctor. He blazes away at a disease where he sees one, as he would at a bear or a lion; the very sight of it excites his organ of destructiveness. Don't you understand me? You hate sin, you know. Well, I hate disease. Moral evil is your devil, and physical evil is mine. I hate it, little or big; I hate to see a fellow sick; I hate to see a child rickety and pale; I hate to see a speck of dirt in the street; I hate to see a woman's gown torn; I hate to see her stockings down at heel; I hate to see anything wasted, anything awry, anything going wrong; I hate to see waterpower wasted, manure wasted, brains wasted; I hate neglect, incapacity, idleness, ignorance, and all the disease and misery which spring out of that. (234)

We move from the explicitly physical domain of disease (the sick fellow) to that of family organization (the rickety child, the torn gown and stockings of the woman) to the larger social issue of waste management and education. Tom is the apostle of order—figured as God's general providence or divine law—in the novel, but even he cannot be truly effective until he realizes his own dependence on something outside of himself. Politics are irrelevant to this social order—it is predicated on the family and the individual body. The law is ineffective, because social change must come through the social and individual organism, not from the state.

GENDER AND SLAVERY

Kingsley's use of slavery as a base metaphor for the social ills he attacks extends throughout his oeuvre. The use of slavery as a metaphor for the plight of British laborers was widespread in the early nineteenth century, as Catherine Gallagher has discussed in detail (*Industrial Reformation*); as she notes, for political radicals, slavery equated to disenfranchisement of the worker (6) and often, a subordination of free will to a deterministic paradigm, and she includes Kingsley's *Alton Locke* in this tradition, as a character torn between these poles, who can finally "individuate" only in his dreams where he is freed from the realm of necessity (Gallagher 101). In *Yeast: A Problem* (1851), the metaphor of slavery is used to represent the effects of the Poor Law, which "suck the independent spirit out of a man" (*Yeast* 231), rather than the condition of the workers. In other words, lack of representation is no longer understood as enslavement, rather, lack of independence is enslavement. This use of slavery as a trope is conventional in this type of literature through the early '50s; however, the direction in which Kingsley takes it in *Two Years Ago* is a new development.

Slavery, a "disease," is like cholera, calling attention to the "sins" and imperfections—usually stemming from selfishness—which must be abjured before a national entity can evolve into its more perfect form. If cholera is the domestic cure for apathy and the selfish refusal to correct "sanitary sins," and the war is explicitly the solution for mid '50s upper-class British men's languid lack of clear direction (*Two Years Ago* 106), the war against slavery is what cements U.S. national identity and also proves the continuity of "English" (British) and U.S. filiation. The novel begins with, and indeed is framed by a discussion of U.S. slavery as moral illness, in a section entitled "Introductory." The conversation that starts the volume, between a British artist, Claude Mellot, and a northern U.S. millionaire, Stangrave, turns on the question of the best method of ending slavery—through war or peaceful means. The American Stangrave pleads, "[Let us] draw a cordon sanitaire round the tainted States, and leave the system to die a natural death, as it rapidly will if it be prevented from enlarging its field" (*Two Years Ago* vi–vii).

U.S. abolition would also wipe out an English sin of the fathers. Kingsley argues in *Westward Ho!*, the 1855 novel of nation building set during the defeat of the Armada and written in part to hearten British soldiers during the Crimean War, that England began to decay morally with its complicity in the American slave trade: the English under Elizabeth are positioned as the enemies of slavery who prevail against the corrupt Spanish slavers. When they see native "slaves" in South America,

> a low murmur of indignation rose from the ambushed Englishmen, worthy of the free and righteous hearts of those days, when Raleigh could appeal to man and God, on the ground of a common humanity, in behalf of the outraged heathens of the New World; when Englishmen still knew that man was man, and that the instinct of freedom was still the righteous voice of God; ere the hapless seventeenth century had brutalised them also, by bestowing on them, amid a hundred other bad legacies, the fatal gift of negro-slaves. (*Westward Ho!* 300)

Interestingly, however, the "slavery" of women *is* required for the project of nation. Having fought the Spanish control of the Americas on the grounds that they enslaved the natives and refused free trade, Amyas comes home to Ayacanora, the Spanish-English woman raised by Native Americans, who pleads, "Only let me fetch and carry for you, tend you, feed you, lead you, like your slave, your dog! Say that I may be your slave!" and more in a like vein. Accepting this rather unorthodox offer of marriage, Amyas lifts her (ambiguously enough, "as the lion lifts the lamb"). The novel ends as she sings a song, "bearing with it the peaceful thoughts of the blind giant back to the Paradises of the West, in the wake of heroes who from that time forth sailed out to colonise another and a vaster England, to the heaven-prospered cry of Westward-Ho!" (413). Women, "naturally" desiring to be slaves, must be used and protected in the relation of marriage, relegated to the noneconomic relationship of home and family, whereas the economic enslavement of laboring men must cease. It is this relationship that supports the ability of men to colonize. Obviously the willing "slavery" of women in marriage is an erotically charged metaphor, whereas the slavery of the natives and Africans in the novel is actual practice. Still, there is a sense that slavery is the natural role of women. The slavery of men, however, in what should be a wage relation (the ownership of one's own body and labor) or the sexual exploitation of women (and perhaps men) undermines nation as it undermines masculinity. These perverse relations, which place what should be familial relations in the economic domain, *are* the principal focus in *Two Years Ago*.

That slavery is ultimately both Britain's curse and its special mission is confirmed by the end of the Marie-Stangrave courtship plot, wherein, just before Tom goes off to the East and Marie and Stangrave become engaged, Tom is hailed by a German policeman who laughs admiringly, "You English! You are all mad, I think! Nothing can shame you, and nothing frighten you! Potz! I believe when your guards at Alma walked into that battery, the other day, every one of them was whistling your Jim Crow, even after he was shot dead!" (*Two Years Ago* 524). It is a peculiar moment in the construction of English identity—first, by a foreigner, second, wherein "Jim Crow" is labeled an English song, rather than an American one. Why of all songs should this be the one under which the British marched to their deaths in the Crimea? The original "Jim Crow" song was popularized in a U.S. minstrel show with white performers in blackface and caught on internationally in the 1830s and '40s—by the '40s, the term had come to mean a black American. It is unclear whether the song alluded to here is the original, or one of the many alternate versions—many of which were abolitionist—which were popularized throughout the century. In any case, however, it is clear that the German envisions the English soldiery going to their deaths whistling a song about American blacks. (Additionally, the reason the German is there at all is that he has been brought to avert a duel between Stangrave and Tom. The hero who brings him is Sabina's "black boy," whose diction places him as an American from the South, probably a freed slave, who is "dancing, grinning, snapping his fingers, in delight at having discovered and prevented the coming tragedy" (524)—the tragedy being that the two white men would waste time fighting each other instead of completing their imperial missions. How the servant comes to do this is never explained.)

The Crimean War and American abolition are thus insistently connected; as in *Westward Ho!*, the English cheerfully die to fight slavery. References to slavery abound in the novel and, as the Crimean War approaches, dovetail with the many references to Eastern Europe, culminating in the Aberalvans refusal to clean up their pigsties, as they wrongly complain of being treated like "Rooshian slave[s]" (301). However, by refusing this imaginary status, they end up being enslaved to "Baalzebub" or cholera, which also stands in for Mammon. In short, each man who refuses to submit himself to a larger cause ends up as a slave to the lower impulses of self. Each woman must "enslave" herself to a man who is worthy of her respect by virtue of his submission to that larger cause in order to *lose* her "hysterical" or "wild" self-devotion, which in Tom's love interest Grace manifests as spiritual pride, sisters Valencia and Lucia as Irish "wildness," and Marie also as "wildness," this time, African.

Marie, the octoroon slave whom Tom buys and then sets free in Canada, decides to become an activist actress, "passing" as an Italian until she has sufficient reputation to pick her own themes and represent the plight of the slave woman on stage. She provides the chivalric quest that will motivate Stangrave to deserve her; she wishes to inspire "a people into manhood" (91). She speaks here of slaves as her people, but earlier she muses on the attractions of white men:

> A slave? Well, what were women meant for but to be slaves? Free them, and they enslave themselves again . . . for they must love. And what blame to them if they love a white man, tyrant though he be, rather than a fellow slave? If the men of our own race will claim us, let them prove themselves worthy of us! Let them rise, exterminate their tyrants, or, failing that, show that they know how to die! Till then, those who are masters of our bodies will be the masters of our hearts. If they crouch before the whites like brutes, what wonder if we look up to him as to a god? Woman must worship, or be wretched. (*Two Years Ago* 90)

For all that Marie fights slavery, it is black men who must rise up against the evil of institutional slavery which weakens American men, especially black men. Until then, she will fight their battles, but this unnatural state of affairs causes her mental strain and leads her to despise the enslaved men she fights for.

Kingsley's women must function as muses, but they are not to act for themselves but to conceive of themselves as worshipers of the men who worship them. Women acting or speaking in the public sphere is a sign of national degeneration, a perversion of woman's true place and a sign of male failure. Therefore, Marie's wildness, as the narrator repeatedly terms it, her impulsiveness, though it is racially defined, is actually a function of her unmarried state, which, in turn, signifies the unworthiness of men to espouse the national cause. Once Stangrave becomes an abolitionist, he marries Marie and all her "wildness" vanishes in an instant. It is through war and in marriage, that men become men, and in the service of a broadly religious conception of a national mission that they become worthy of women. Moral wars secure empire, and it is through this Christian soldierdom that men are masculinized.

NATION AND FEMININITY

Nation, then, is emphatically the business of men, to be enacted upon and through the bodies of women, but not by them. Unlike Kingsley's other novels featuring epidemic disease, there is little call for social work on the part of women in *Two Years Ago*—the religious enthusiast Grace prays with the sick, and nurses and educates children, but she is powerless to enact sanitary reform against the prejudice of the Aberalvans. Despite Kingsley's long-standing commitment to medical training of women and encouragement of women to do sanitary work, the other women in his novels never dream of doing sanitary work; that is the work of men. Even in *Yeast*, wherein women are encouraged by other characters to do sanitary work, the heroine Argemone dies in the attempt and her sister Honoria contracts a wasting disease, which keeps her housebound. Women suffer for the sins of men, but cannot themselves atone for them. In the moment of crisis, the social is fully masculinized as the substratum of nation in this novel, and the role of women then becomes purely inspirational, to motivate men to take up causes, causes which are national but narrated in terms of women's sexual exploitation, and then to worship them when they do. Marie, of course, takes up the abolitionist cause, but repeatedly bemoans that she must do so because American men are not living up to their responsibilities; once Stangrave does, she retires into private life.

What is wrong with England and the United States is figured, like slavery, as a sexual scandal. Once again, unlike earlier novels wherein capitalism was the target of Kingsley's critique, here slavery is taken out of an economic context and into a domestic and sexual one.[3] Further, the English characters come to grief, not through financial woes, as in so many narratives of the 1840s and '50s, but through sexual jealousy (as does Vavasour) and other forms of physical intemperance, usually addiction. Those characters who have been redeemed are rescued from sexually questionable pasts. Sabina, who is hinted to have been a fallen woman, exchanges the story of her own life for Marie's recounting of her enslavement; that it is the sensational story of a woman's sexual exploitation is repeatedly invoked by the novel that cannot or will not recount the story: "What it was need not be told. A little common sense, and a little knowledge of human nature, will enable the reader to fill up for himself the story of a beautiful slave" (*Two Years Ago* 146). Marie finds "a sister in the communion of sorrows" in Sabina (146). The reader—here explicitly male—will know; for the unmarried woman, it is better not to.

Tom himself is briefly enslaved in Circassia, and "very nearly . . . sold for slaves into Persia, which would not have been pleasant" before he escapes (14). In turn, he has agreed to go to the U.S. South to try to free a slave girl there who is the beloved of a dead comrade, a goal in which all of his English friends concur, seeing her slavery there entirely in terms of sexual degradation. The laconic reference to the peculiarities of male Persian slavery—as "not pleasant," in comparison to the mere beatings, imprisonment, and dirty work that the Tartars' enslavement imposes, is indicated in the characters' unwillingness to define the exact urgency behind rescuing the slave girl, explained in terms of the presence of a young girl at the discussion: "'no one shall say that . . . he let a poor girl—' and recollecting Mary's presence, he finished his sentence by sundry stamps and thumps of the table" (*Two Years Ago* 15).

It is perhaps stretching a point to observe that this discussion of sexual exploitation gestures toward Tom's danger in the Persian bazaar—and that what causes him to "lose his nerve" finally is eighteen months in a Turkish prison, both regions included in what Burton would call the Sotadic zone in 1888 (Sedgwick 183). Only Grace (that is, marriage to Grace Harvey) enables him to regain this phallus of which the continual threat of decapitation in the prison has robbed him. In any case, sexual violation is, directly for women, and at least metonymically for men (through various violations of the body's integrity) that which destroys the tissue of national cohesiveness. Kingsley indicates in a letter that Tom's "temptation" is sexual:

> men of his character (like all strong men till God's grace takes hold of them) are weak upon one point . . . —everything they can stand but that; and the more they restrain themselves from prudential motives, the more sudden and violent is the temptation when it comes. I have indicated as delicately as I could the world-wide fact, which all know and all ignore; had I not done so, Thurnall would have been a chimaera fit only for a young lady's novel. (*Letters and Memories* 58)

The reference is somewhat ambiguous. It may refer to his near-assault on Grace, and possibly to past liaisons with women, which are hinted at in various points in the novel, however, the ultimate temptation or trial that he undergoes—which breaks him—is in the Turkish prison. Also, mere rakishness seems hardly to fit the description of "the world-wide fact, which all know and all ignore." For Kingsley, nation must be predicated on the integrity of the male body, men's ownership of their own labor, and freedom to exchange it. It is further guaranteed by the protection of women whose sexuality is contained within marriage and who produce, in turn, manly men. England, which succumbs to the lure of slavery, the dependence on a feminized black male labor force during the seventeenth century, will not be truly free of this original sin at the heart of modernity until the United States abolishes slavery and England secures and "civilizes" her colonies and trade routes in the East.

This theme is reinforced in *Two Years Ago*. Slavery in this novel, as is often the case in British abolition literature, means less forced labor than sexual exploitation. Lavington, the ancestral squire of Whitbury, the quintessentially English town in Berkshire where the framing narrative begins, has died without issue and been replaced in the people's affections by the more democratic Carlylean hero, Mark Armsworth, the town banker and sanitary housing reformer. Later, we discover that Marie, the octoroon slave girl whom Mark helps to free and who claims she has the blood of a good English family in her veins, is also named Lavington. The Lavingtons come from the same area in Berkshire where the Stangraves come from; the American millionaire Stangrave discovers that in marrying Marie and taking up the cause of abolition, he is avenging the wrongs as well as atoning for the sins of his family's neighbors and perhaps, relatives. The end of the "Introductory" section gives the reader a legend for reading the text: the novel consists of "facts, which shall be duly set forth in this tale, saving and excepting, of course, the real reason why everybody did everything. For . . . the true springs of all human action are generally those which fools will not see, which wise men will not mention: so that, in order to present a readable tragedy of Hamlet, you must 'always omit the part of Hamlet,'—and probably the ghost and the queen into the bargain" (xxiii).

Other than a joke on the complexity of human motivations, we see that the unrepresentable matter here is sex and sexual shame, fratricide and fraternal usurpation. The economic and sexual selfishness at the heart of slavery is the same set of motivations that lead to all the "sins" in the novel, the solution for which is a spiritual regeneration which cannot take place without a recognition of the interconnectedness of the social body. This interconnectedness is denied when the characters refuse to acknowledge and impose order on the "unspeakable" aspects of bodily experience—illicit sexuality, bodily wastes, and so forth. Again and again, the text will draw close to the matter of sexual abuse, and coyly refuse to detail it—in a manner that makes it impossible to misunderstand. The other material treated this way is, of course, human waste, which Kingsley refers to as "that which we euphemize as decaying organic matter" or "id genus omne," and the symptoms of cholera, which prompt the narrator to "draw a veil over the too dreadful" details. ("Id genus omne" here refers to sewage, but it classically refers to death—also "that which is common to all.") Kingsley is writing a book centered around those bodily happenings that cannot be narrated. It is such haunting unrepresentability that is indicated by Queen Gertrude and, perhaps, the ancient complicity of Britain in slavery that is the other ghost demanding exorcism through justice.

Two Years Ago is a sequel to *Yeast*, Kingsley's earlier sanitary novel, and continues with the characters and themes of that novel. It is in *Yeast* that the story of the amusingly named Lavingtons, ancestors of Marie, is told, and there it is both a sanitary and sexual sin that the Lavingtons are cursed for. The curse goes back to the dispossession of nuns from the estate (homage here to Disraeli's *Sybil*, in which the role of dispossessed Catholic abbeys is also significant as a national sin to be expiated). But more significantly, though the prioress curses the Lavingtons for the dispossession, the unforgivable act happened afterward: "he [the Squire] or his . . . that night, said something or did something to the lady, that was more than woman's heart could bear: and the next morning, she was found dead and cold, drowned in that weir-pool [the Nun-pool]" and all the heirs since have drowned there (*Yeast* 261). The curse, it is said, will not be lifted until the water runs uphill, from the Nun-pool to Ashy Down: that is, until sanitary irrigation overcomes the evils of human injustice. With questionable justice, the curse extends to the villagers, who will continue to degenerate until the curse is lifted, thus driving home the point that, although the responsibility lies with the ruling classes, the social body is a unity and suffers as one.

That the "something" done by Squire Lavington or his men is a rape is strongly indicated not only by the language, but by the fact that the Lavington curse that Kingsley bases his fictional story on was actually rooted in the "seduction" of a village girl in the eighteenth century; the legend has it that the Lavingtons were cursed by her father (Chapman 91). But Kingsley modifies the tale to make a woman the origin of the curse, and perhaps thus underscores the curse's nature as linked to the violation of chastity rather than of property. Further, the ballad that precipitates the fall of the family in the novel connects the poor sanitary condition of the workers, the decadent and vicious condition of the ruling classes, and especially the sexual abuse of the village women: "our daughters with base-born babes / Have wandered away in their shame / If your misses had slept, squire, where they did / Your misses might do the same" (*Yeast* 204). The squire, upon being confronted with this ballad, has an apoplectic fit. His two daughters die, one of typhus caught in laborers' cabins, and the other of a wasting disease. The heir, of course, has already drowned in the Nun-pool, so the family dies out entirely, making way for the reign of the banker who is the pillar of the town in *Two Years Ago*. As the protagonist's love interest, Argemone, dies, she suffers from a persistent scent-memory of the filth of the cottages, and says that "the curse of the Lavingtons had truly come upon her. To perish by the people whom they made. . . . There are those horrible scents again! . . . The Nun-pool! Take all the water, every drop, and wash Ashy clean. . . . Make a great fountain in it . . . to wash away the sins of the Lavingtons" (*Yeast* 330).[4]

Two Years Ago continues *Yeast's* connection between sexual exploitation of women and sanitary neglect. In place of concern with the economic situation of the laborers, however, we have the need to aggressively rule and defend empire and the abolition of slavery in the United States. Nation is still built by the expiation of sexual abuse, the imposition of sanitary order on the domestic social body and the abolition of slavery. *Yeast* ends with the heroes beginning a journey of discovery to the land of Prester John, a place where the "body and the spirit . . . are no longer separate" (347), a "Caucasian Utopia." This journey, like those seen in *Alton Locke* and *Hypatia*, begins in Asia, but must ultimately end in building a "Caucasian empire" (347)—explicitly to be realized by Britain, its white colonies, and the United States. Still, it is significant that the country of Prester John that is the utopian referent is the old legend of a utopian Christian community that was used during the Crusades to urge resistance to the expanding Turkish empire. The imposition of Christian—and here, explicitly Caucasian ideals—in the East was a powerful legitimation for the expansion of exploratory and imperialist activities from West to East. It is this set of tasks that is taken up in *Two Years Ago*.

Like Tom, the United States is overly proud of its self-sufficiency, and attributes that to its own efforts; Tom infuriates Stangrave by making the economic argument that America's success is based on an accident of geography and the wealth of land "Westward Ho" at Americans' disposal. In a key passage, Tom poses a central question of the constitution of nation: "Do you mean by America, the country, or the people? You boast, all of you, of your country, as though you made it yourselves; and quite forget that God made America, and America has made you" (*Two Years Ago* 434). The land's ownership is a historical accident; the people are the true nation, and Stangrave's definition of the American man leaves out a significant number of "men and brothers." When Stangrave argues, "The glory of America is, that . . . the man . . . is too well fed, too prosperous, too well educated to be made a slave of," Tom responds, "And therefore makes slaves of the niggers instead? . . . I shan't believe in that [American moral superiority] while I see the whole of the northern states so utterly given up to the "almighty dollar" that they leave the honor of their country to be made ducks and drakes of by a few southern slaveholders" (*Two Years Ago* 434).

Stangrave, upon consideration, also accuses America of a national self-aggrandizement: "The old Jew used to say of his nation. 'It is God that has made us, and not we ourselves.' We say, 'It is we that have made ourselves, while God—?'" He muses that Calvinism has failed to consider "the bodies and the national future of the whole negro race" while saving individual souls (436). Whereas Britain grew, as Stangrave muses, "like Topsy" (!), the United States started on principles of equality that have been violated from the outset; it is the original sin that taints "God's new Eden" (435). If Britain is the slave child that muddles along toward freedom without a plan, the United States is more culpable in having deliberately abdicated the responsibilities of freedom: "White slaves? We, perhaps, and not the English peasant are the white slaves!" (435). War, he concludes, may be necessary. Close upon his identification of the United States with the chosen nation, he runs into a German Jew who says he has seen Marie and mistook her for Jewish, "one of the Nation" (439). Nation can only be constructed around the avowal of the rights and needs of bodies that have been excluded from consideration; the "national" future of the "negro race" is the American national future, just as control of the disavowed products and needs of the wayward working-class body that has "just growed"—and overgrown its bounds—are necessary for Britain. These bodies, in turn, must be inscribed and transformed by the national narrative.

INSCRIBING NATION ON THE BODY

Just as nations are based upon and constituted from individual bodies, such bodies bear the imprint of national narratives, and can be altered by them. In Kingsley's parable of bodily and national interdependence, evolution is not only potentially multidirectional, but immediately transformative. Like *Water Babies*, Kinglsey's 1863 parable of spiritual and hygienic growth for children, *Two Years Ago* is preoccupied with the theme of spiritual evolution. Kingsley also develops here the idea of multiple evolutions on different planes of existence, comparing humans to insects and sea creatures who go through radical metamorphoses yet remain the same creature. This evolution can also take place, to a lesser extent, within a lifetime, in which it is possible for people to become more purely themselves. Sin is figured as marks and scars on the surface of character, and scarring plays an important role in the novel's vision of spiritual development. Marie, hearing of Sabina's difficult history, marvels, "And you have been through all this, so beautiful and bright as you are . . . yet not a scar or a wrinkle has it left behind" to which Sabina replies, "they were there once, Marie; but God and Claude smoothed them away" (*Two Years Ago* 146).

Tom, like all Kingsley's heroes, has a flaw, and it is precisely the ungodliness of absolute self-sufficiency that is both the ideal and limit of the Kingsley man:

> Tom was now . . . an altogether accomplished man of the world. . . . He had to use men, and, therefore to watch how he used them; to watch every word, gesture, tone of voice and, in all times and places, do the fitting thing. It was hard work; but necessary for a man who stood alone and self-poised in the midst of the universe; fashioning for himself everywhere, just as far as his arm could reach, some not intolerable condition, depending on nothing but himself. (*Two Years Ago* 20–21)

Unlike all the other characters, who rely on hysteria, doctrinal authority, drugs, alcohol, or other outside sources of stimulants, Tom is a self-contained system. But this, too, although superior to the other male characters, is finally inadequate. Man's incompleteness must be supplemented with service to humanity and faith in God, and women's with faith in man, through whom she experiences faith in God. If other characters sense their incompleteness too poignantly, Tom's "disease" is that he fails to even realize the incompleteness that is a necessary component of his humanity.

Tom also fails to believe either in divine punishment or in the evolution toward some higher state of being, which he considers a threat to his identity: he "would be sorry" to change, for "Thomas Thurnall is an old friend. . . . I should be sorry to lose his company" (343). The exemplary Major Campbell, veteran of Indian service and voice of true religion in the novel, asks him,

> "What if those points [flaws] were not really any part of your character, but mere excrescences of disease; or, if that be too degrading a notion, mere scars of old wounds, and of the wear and tear of life; what if, in some future life, all those disappeared, and the true Thomas Thurnall, pure and simple, were alone left? . . . what if that self-conceit and self-dependence were the very root of all the disease, the cause of all the scars, the very thing that will have to be got rid of, before our true character and true manhood can be developed?" . . . [But the major] knew that with such men words are of little avail. The disease was intrenched too strongly in the very centre of the man's being. (*Two Years Ago* 343–44)

Here again, then we have "scars" caused by "disease" that are mistaken for essential components of character, much like Sabina's scars, or Marie's racial attributes that can be removed through spiritual renewal.

As is typical in Kingsley novels, this self-assertiveness of the hero must be broken. Interestingly, however, unlike other novels wherein this breakdown is lovingly detailed (such as Amyas's blinding in *Westward Ho!*), in *Two Years Ago*, it happens offstage: we are merely told of it secondhand. Tom goes off after the cholera epidemic to do secret service work in Russia but ends up in a Turkish prison before the action even starts:

> shut up by a mistake!—at the very outset, too!—by a boorish villain of a khan, on a drunken suspicion;—a fellow whom I was trying to serve. . . . I was caught in my own trap! I went out full blown with self-conceit. . . . And this brute to stop me short—to . . . keep me there eighteen months threatening to cut of my head once a quarter. . . . I found out that I had been trying for years which was the stronger, God or I; I found out I had been trying whether I could not do well enough without Him; and there I found I could not. (*Two Years Ago* 540)

He says he has lost his "nerve." I hardly dare stir about now, lest some harm should come to me" (540). Through the loss of his freedom, a recapitulation of the Persian slavery he escapes earlier, he finds the limits of self-reliance, just as, through the humiliating defeats in the Crimea, including the decimation of the army by cholera, the aimless British male characters find a purpose and seriousness that saves them and prepares them for marriage.[5]

And so, the narrator states in the last line of the novel, as Grace agrees to marry Tom, "the old heart passed away" and he gets a new one (540), much as Marie's "theatric passionateness" (a trait Kingsley persistently associates with her African blood) "had passed;—'Nothing was left of her, / Now, but pure womanly,'" the minute she accepts Stangrave's proposal (527). Although earlier we were told unequivocally that Marie had "the strange double nature which so many Quadroons seem to owe to their mixed blood; a strong side of deep feeling, ambition, energy, an intellect rather Greek in its rapidity than English in sturdiness; and withal a weak side, of instability . . . sometimes, too, a tendency to untruth, which is the mark, not perhaps of the African specially, but of every enslaved race" (147), here these racial characteristics become inessential "scars" that can be erased through spiritual evolution; these racial characteristics are also here read as the result of slavery, even though elsewhere Kingsley appears to enact a wavering commitment to at least a geographic essentialism.

NATION AND RACIAL TRANSFORMATION

Kingsley's character Claude Mellot, an artist, in a discussion of realism in painting, suggests that, in Marie's face in repose or

> in deep thought, there are lines in it which utterly puzzle one,—touches which are eastern, Kabyle, almost Quadroon. . . . But who sees them in the light of that beauty? They are defects, no doubt, but defects which no one would observe without a deep study of the face. They express her character no more than a scar would; and therefore when I paint her . . . I shall utterly ignore them. If, on the other hand, I met the same lines in a face which I knew to have Quadroon blood in it, I should religiously copy them; because then they would be integral elements of the face. (*Two Years Ago* 144)

The reference to the Kabyle, an Afro-Semitic people from the Mahgreb, strengthens the reference to the Jews (though the Kabyle are Muslim). So race is in the eye of the beholder, as well as the flesh of the beheld; the "truth" of the face that can be portrayed in painting depends on what one "knows to be true."

One might see this as a critique of the biologism of race, and so, in part is it meant, as Kingsley shows when he suggests that character traits associated with "Africanness" may be the result of slavery. Yet, Claude does see those traits there because they are actually there, and, indeed, Claude gives up painting in favor of photography later in the novel because of its superior accuracy or truthfulness: positivism with a vengeance (265). He does so, despite the fact that at an earlier time he derides photography as unable to capture the truth of the face as we see it—a constantly mobile and expressive surface inflected with the movement and memories of the observer (143). That Kingsley's racial and geographic politics are confused is hardly news; most of his critics have found them baffling. However, a few persistent lines of thought emerge in this novel, which, like Kingsley's other novels, are centrally concerned with issues of national identity, and racial and ethnic mixing.

If the scars of "worldliness" are part of an inauthentic self, a disease, which are wiped away by religion, the status of race in its relation to nation is more problematic. Marie's scars and other bodily traces of her racial identity, which, when believed to be inauthentic, are discussed as scars by Claude Mellot, threaten to become all encompassing when the woman bears the burden of the battle for nation. Once the burden is transferred to the man, the scars fade away into "pure" womanliness (which, it seems, is white). Until then, Marie is the avatar of (every) nation: America in Stangrave's liberty plays, the African American "nation" and the Jewish diaspora (for a German Jewish character). Marie herself connects the plight of her people to that of Italy—also struggling for nationhood and unification—and takes an Italian name to hide her identity and to legitimate her concern with portraying issues of liberty and democracy on stage, and later, Tom, who liberated Marie, will be mistaken by a German policeman for Italian nationalist Giuseppe Mazzini. Afterward, she moves offstage to raise her children, apparently in contented domesticity, having given up her passion for reform to Stangrave, who takes up the cause in her stead.

However, we also know that if Mellot knew Marie to be an octoroon, he would paint her that way as part of the "truth" of her identity, whereas, as it is, her occasionally African or "Eastern" expression is simply a "flaw" like a "scar"—wiped away apparently by the development into a more advanced phase of existence, as Tom's development is compared, in one of the persistent evolutionary and natural history metaphors of the novel, to the emergence of a mollusk from a larval to a mature form. In marrying Stangrave and producing children, Marie becomes the avatar of a new hybrid nation but is simultaneously "purified" of her Africanness and duality. Race, then, though Tom believes it to be basic to the limit of "moral development" is actually a "scar" or flaw, something inauthentic to personhood and nationhood that are essentially deracinated, where deracination means something very like an "Aryan"

(*Alton Locke*) or "Caucasian" (*Yeast*) Englishness. At the same time, the traits
of theatricality associated with Marie's "wild Tropic blood" are ambiguously
represented as essential (blood), geographical (Tropic), and the product of
slavery, while the emotionalistic traits of the many Irish characters in the novel
(the Scoutbush/St. Just family) are seemingly immutably rooted in racial identity. (The Welsh, however, dark as they are, are presented squarely and repeatedly as examples of the "English character.")

There are also real scars left by slavery that cannot be erased, but can be
transformed into an inspirational text. Stangrave and Marie marry when he
agrees to take over her quest: "'I will not fail or falter, till I have won justice
for you and your race. . . . I will prize them [the scars left by the whip on
Marie's back] . . . more than all your loveliness. I will see in them God's com-
mandment to me, written not on tables of stone, but on fair, pure, noble flesh.
My Marie! You shall have cause even to rejoice in them!'" (*Two Years Ago* 527).
Here the scars that are immutable are transformed into the sign of God's com-
mandment toward nationhood; at the same time, the reminders of Marie's
"race" are written on "fair" flesh. Interestingly, the protean Marie, who stands
for every oppressed nation, loses this protean quality—and, in fact, any ability
to represent nation at all, becoming "pure womanly" at the moment Stangrave
accepts the Quest. She then immediately goes literally offstage, and is eliminated from the novel as an active character. However, blackness is feminized
here and black nationhood made a white man's burden.

Kingsley's thoughts on race changed radically over the course of the mid-
century, as did many of his peers.' By the mid-1860s, he was supporting the
repressive activities of Governor Eyre in Jamaica (as in the '50s, he had supported Rajah Brooke of Sarawak). By this time, he had not only utterly repudiated his Chartist-era support for manhood suffrage, but also his position on
the potential equality of races: "I held that doctrine [of natural human equal-
ity] strongly myself in past years, and was cured of it . . . by the harsh school
of facts. . . . I have seen, also, that the differences of race are so great, that certain races, e.g., the Irish Celts, seem quite unfit for self-government" (*Life and
Works* 2: 226). However, he goes on to indicate that education and religion
may also play a role (Catholic nations, he suggests, are stunted). In fact, as
early as 1850, Kingsley is embracing the Teutonism that Carlyle popularized
in the '40s; this can easily be seen in the evolutionary narrative of the dream
sequence in *Alton Locke*, and later in *Hypatia* (1853), as literary scholar
Stephen Prickett notes (67–68).

Yet the strict racializing and biologizing of those traits comes even later
in Kingsley than it does for many mid-Victorian thinkers. For most Victorians, race was still an unclear mixture of biology, ethnic heritage, and geographic location.[6] It is probably not accidental that recourse to a more essen-
tialized vision of racial difference along American lines becomes attractive to

British thinkers in the years immediately following the 1857 war in India. In *Yeast*, published in 1847, Kingsley privileges race mixing as a mode to achieve a healthfulness that is quintessentially "Norse," and derides theories of essential racial difference:

> How classic, how independent of clime or race is its [the hero Tregarva's face's] bland, majestic, self-possession! How thoroughly Norse its massive squareness! . . . Like all noble races, the Cornish owe their nobleness to the impurity of their blood—to its perpetual loans from foreign veins. See how the serpentine curve of his nose, his long nostril, and protruding, sharp-cut lips, mark his share of Phoenician or Jewish blood! How Norse, again, that dome-shaped forehead! How Celtic, those dark curls, that restless grey eye . . . like Von Troneg Hagen's in the Niebelungen Lied. (70)

The protagonist considers local workers "rather a degraded than an undeveloped race" having large brain cases unlike the "Kabyle" but "loose and sensual lower features"—drawing on the popular notion of skull shape as racially essential and connected to intelligence, but facial features as showing the effects of environment. But he is immediately rebuked for "jumbling . . . the 'physical understanding' of the brain, with the 'pure intellect' of the spirit" (*Yeast* 241) and told to mark instead the effects of degeneration within the community caused by poor sanitary conditions, poor diet, and vice. The pure intellect, it seems, is very much affected by physical environment. What we still see in *Two Years Ago* is racial and geographical and experiential traits all combining, without a clear sense of the priority of any of the categories, to produce an organism who can *then* be typed along a developmental and evolutionary progression toward an ideal embodied by a certain ethnic type. Further, it is possible for individuals, at least to a certain extent, to evolve in their own bodies toward the Teutonic ideal.

Perhaps the last word on racial—again blending into geographical—typing in *Two Years Ago* is in the description of Tardrew, the surly overseer, who refuses to update the cottages on the estate he manages, loses his daughter to the cholera, and then manages to admit that the surgeon was right:

> By those curt and surly utterances did Tardrew, in true British Bulldog fashion, express a repentance too deep for words; too deep for all confessionals, penances, and emotions or acts or contrition; the repentance not of the excitable and theatric southern, unstable as water, even in his most violent remorse; but of the still, deep-hearted northern, whose pride breaks slowly and silently, but breaks once for all; who tells to God what he will never tell to man; and, having told it, is a new creature from that day forth forever. (352)

In an evolutionary paradigm, the "southern" person, "unstable as water," is able to evolve quickly and easily because she or he is more open, fluid, and unstable—at an early phase of evolution as an organism or individual and therefore more clearly a collection of tissues to be transformed rapidly. However, the southerner can also degenerate quickly. The imperial "northern," more closed, individual, and hard-set, is also harder to transform, but when the transformation happens, it is more permanent.

Thus we see explained Marie's strange racial fluidity; when she dreads the revelation of her African identity to Stangrave, she experiences a hallucination of racial degeneration:

> as she looked [in the mirror]—was it the mere play of her excited fancy,—or did her eyelid slope more and more, her nostrils shorten and curl, her lips enlarge, her mouth itself protrude? It was more than the play of fancy: for Stangrave saw it as well as she. Her actress's imagination, fixed on the African type with an intensity proportioned to her dread of seeing it in herself, had moulded her features. . . . Another half minute, and that face had melted out of the mirror as well, at least for Marie's eyes; and in its place an ancient negress, white-haired, withered as the wrinkled ape, but with eyes closed in death . . . to that old dame's coffin had her mother, the gay quadroon woman, flaunting in finery which was the price of shame, led Marie . . . and call[ed] it her dear old granny. (*Two Years Ago* 138)

Again, this remarkable fluidity is fixed once Marie accepts Stangrave's offer of marriage.

Thus, although "developmental" characteristics are mapped onto geography and, to some extent, race, they are simultaneously de-essentialized. Kingsley also insistently and deliberately includes Irish, Scottish, Welsh, English, Anglo-American, and African American characters, all of whom are sometimes described in terms of "national" traits, but all of whom also reveal alliances with other nations. (The African American woman is also of English blood, as is the Anglo-American. The Welshmen are quintessentially English, and the Scotsman is the spiritual ideal of the English characters. The artist who represents the "English point of view" in the introduction is named Claude Mellot and is married to an exotic, slightly Eastern beauty.) These diverse characters share an eclectic mix of religious beliefs (Anglican, Methodist, Irish Protestant, agnostic, mystic). Kingsley thus moves away from an essential view of identity, as he also does by presenting the marriage of the "mixed blood" woman to the white American as the triumphant end of their love story.

C. J. W. L. Wee argues that "The difference from the modern he [Kingsley] proposes requires a recuperation of primitive energy now vanished from England; at the same time, racial purity, even at a strictly literary-cultural level, must be maintained, even though barbarous energy can only be found in imperial frontier territories" (68). Wee also notes that Lamarckian evolution is important to Kingsley's vision of national identity, but fails to mark the changing notion of racial biologism that informs Kingsley's work over the mid-century, and is unable to account for the major inconsistencies in Kingsley's theories of racial purity, despite having the key to them in the evolutionary dream he retells from *Alton Locke*: racial traits *evolve*, for Kingsley. The "primitive vigor" of the Other that the Englishman must recoup is in fact his own primitive vigor, attenuated by culture, but still present in the body's evolutionary past. When Eleanor exhorts the tailor-poet Alton Locke to go to the tropics for inspiration and thus restore jaded English literature, she is asking him to be as other colonizers, like "the conquerors of Hindostan." This will enable the working classes who read it to "claim their share in a national life," necessary because "the nation is a spiritual body" (Kingsley in Wee 73). Wee finds all of this an odd prescription for reviving Teutonic vigor, but if spiritual evolution enables one to become more oneself, the only kind of vigor that can be expressed in a unified English (British) nation *is* Teutonic—whatever its origins, that will be its expression in the organism.[7]

NATION AND CHOLERA

If the slavery narrative provides the overarching logic of the story in *Two Years Ago*, the cholera epidemic is the climax of the novel, bringing several of the storylines together (though it exempts the American characters, whose battles are not to be fought in that arena, reinforcing the logic of the novel that assigns tasks by nation: abolition to the Americans, sanitation and control of the East to the British). Despite Kingsley's scientific rhetoric, the arrival of the cholera in Aberalva is figured, if not as divine retribution, in terms reminiscent of religious explanations of the plague:

> He had come at last,—Baalzebub, god of flies, and of what flies are bred from,—to visit his self-blinded worshippers, and bestow on them his own Cross of the Legion of Dishonour. He had come suddenly, capriciously, sportively, as he sometimes comes. . . . He fleshes his teeth on every kind of prey. The drunken cobbler dies, of course; but spotless cleanliness and sobriety does not save the mother of seven children, who has been soaking her brick floor daily with water from a poisoned well, defiling where she meant to clean. (*Two Years Ago* 320)

Yet Kingsley also takes advantage of the occasion to critique what he sees as extremist religious attitudes toward the cholera, and to disassociate the established church from those positions. After the first wave of deaths caused by sanitary reasons, comes a wave of deaths caused by panic exacerbated by a preacher who has come to the town to get up a revival. (He frightens three women into dying of cholera the first day.) The major goes to challenge the preacher, and is so filled with the holy spirit himself that he demands an accounting for the deaths of the "innocent souls to whom you have slandered their heavenly Father by your devil's doctrines this day. . . . Let the Lord judge between you and me. He knows best how to make his judgment manifest" (*Two Years Ago* 330). In a rare post–Old Testament intervention, the Lord obligingly strikes the preacher with cholera on the spot: "In two hours he was blue; in four he was dead. The judgment, as usual, had needed no miracle to enforce it" (*Two Years Ago* 331). Kingsley accedes to the doctrine of special providence by denying it, and by implication critiques the opposition using their main premise. God, here, is able to show his will through direct intervention, which is "no miracle" because it follows directly from the General Providence of natural law.

Each character is tainted in some way, and that taint is both represented by and comes to crisis in fighting the cholera. Those who are beyond help are generally represented as addicts. Like slave owners, they rely on something outside of themselves for their existence, yet it is something subordinate to themselves, instead of, as it should be, an overarching sense of Christian community and purpose. However, for those who do not die, the cholera provides a chance for spiritual renewal through suffering. For Frank, who works hard for his parishioners, the cholera is a rite of passage. Happy to have become ill in the service of his religion and looking forward to escaping a hopeless love, Frank, "just as he was making a man," as Tom laments, ends up "screaming like a woman, though he has bitten his tongue half through to stop his screams" (*Two Years Ago* 338). He recovers, however, declares his love for Lord Scoutbush's sister, wins her hand, and goes to fight in the Crimea, returning to his curacy afterward with the hard-won support of the entire village of tough-minded, largely Methodist fishermen. Kingsley is insistent in his scientific reasoning, and also on his refusal to attribute cholera to God's wrath—having God show his wrath in earnest by killing the itinerant preacher with cholera for saying that God sent the cholera in the first place. Still, as this example suggests, the status of the cholera as the wages of sin is ambiguous. It can have a tonic effect on the morally flawed. Also, though the innocent die with the guilty, the guilty are picked out for special mention and their vulnerability to cholera is explicitly connected to their sins.

Cholera, then, bodies forth what is wrong with the English individually (their self-centeredness, "effeminate" weakness), as the war does nationally (their lack of overarching moral purpose), while simultaneously providing a purifying challenge that will result in evolutionary change, both personal and national, in the survivors. Those who are not suffering from this form of weakness, such as Tom, who has had cholera twice in the course of his travels and so does not fear it (*Two Years Ago* 69), are reserved to be "cured" by the war. This evolution is tied to the renewal and development of nation; as the artist Claude Mellot says in the "Introductory" chapter, what followed from 1855 is that "a spirit of self-reform has been awakened round here, in many a heart I thought was utterly frivolous. In fine, in every circle of every class, men and women are asking to be taught their duty, that they may go and do it; I find everywhere schools, libraries and mechanics institutes" and material improvements (ix). His interlocutor, Stangrave, accredits this to

> that belief in God's being, in some mysterious way, the living King of England and of Christendom [which] . . . has led you to *reform*, as brave strong men should dare to do; a people who have been for many an age in the vanguard of all the nations, and the champions of sure and solid progress throughout the world; because what is new among you is not patched artificially on to the old, but grows organically out of it, with a growth like that of your own English oak, whose every new-year's leaf-crop is fed by roots which burrow deep in many a buried generation, and the rich soil of full a thousand years. (*Two Years Ago* ix)

Reform, then, is tissue regeneration on a national scale, but it can only come out of a deeply rooted national past—a regeneration that is not alien to the individual but emerges from its very sources of identity.

For all his commitment to science, which is abundantly clear throughout the novel in its allusions to the importance of chemistry, natural history, and up-to-date tissue theory, Kingsley is solidly sanitarian. The cholera in this novel is not contagious; it is a filth disease born in part of an epidemic constitution. Perhaps what this illustrates most clearly is the way that the medical and sanitary views overlapped in the public mind by the mid-century and before the widespread acceptance of John's Snow waterborne theory; after Chadwick, there was no need for a clear distinction politically and many laypeople and medics understood the disease through some combination of theories. Tom's is the voice of medical (and sanitary) reason in the novel—up to a point. But Kingsley's fascination with evolution (he himself said the novel was about "self-evolution" (*Life and Works* 3: 40) and medical-histological theory is also evident in the character of Campbell, the natural historian and advocate of spiritual evolution, and of Stangrave, whose "metaphysics," as the narrator calls them, are taken in large part from popular understanding of Bichat (though the narrator attributes them only to Emerson and Fuller). Stangrave muses that the river, may be but a collection of ever changing atoms of water;—what is your body but a similar collection of atoms, decaying and renewing every moment? Yet you are a person; and is not the river, too, a person—a live thing? It has an individual countenance which you love, which you would recognize again, meet it where you will; it marks the whole landscape; it determines probably, the geography and the society of a whole district. (*Two Years Ago* x)

This comment, in the "Introductory" section of the novel, is in part a response to the cleansing of the polluted river over the two years since the epidemic, and celebration of sanitary reform. But it also introduces the theme of physical (tissue) regeneration through physical evolution that plays out in the discussion of the erasure of scars and that holds an important role in Kingsley's religious beliefs. The river is cleansed, but it is still the same river and still has the same recognizable essence; it is only the impurities, inessential to its character, that have washed away, leaving the same "individual," the same "person." Despite being made of tissues, decaying and renewing constantly, somehow, those individual "atoms" make up an individual, a person;[8] as Bichat would say, it has both organic and animal life. Tom, however, despite his Paris training (which in this period would have exposed him to Bichat's ideas) and his love of microscopes, is an old-fashioned medic, who finally recognizes only the level of the individual organism, and is distrustful of change or evolution as a process that impinges on the "animal" life, the self as a whole, rather than the "organic" level of tissue.

But Kingsley recuperates Bichat in the service of, as he calls it, metaphysics. Whereas Bichat emphasized the death process—contending that life was a constant battle against dying tissues the organism eventually lost—Kingsley focuses on the death of tissue as a means for regeneration of the organism. In a Spencerian move, he sees the cholera as the cleansing of weak tissue and the opportunity to regenerate damaged tissue of the social body, though he focuses more on the victims' potential for spiritual renewal than on the elimination of the unfit. And when Tom accepts that he is not sufficient unto himself, an organic whole that is a closed system, the "breakdown" precipitates new development that enables his "old heart to pass away, and instead of it grew up a heart like his father's, even the heart of a little child," in the line that concludes the novel (540). Though the boyishness and character flaws of several of the characters (Scoutbush, Trebooze) are wiped away in the war, where the threat of the body's violent dissolution lends them seriousness and purpose, Tom, the already manly veteran of many wars with no strong national allegiances, is broken of his rational individualism by the *containment* of his body and becomes "as a child" again, much as Tardrew becomes "a new creature," or Sabine's scars and wrinkles are wiped away.

In other words, Tom must accept the interdependence of man and God, but also of individuals with each other, and the openness of a system in which the individual can only retain a living personhood by allowing parts of himself to be defined as inessential, to be cleansed away, like the emergence of an adult insect from a larval form (*Two Years Ago* 343). In 1862, Kingsley writes in a letter to biologist and professor George Rolleston: "the soul of each living being down to the lowest, secretes the body thereof . . . the body is nothing more than the expression in terms of matter, of the stage of development to which the being has arrived . . . I wish you would envisager [*sic*] that gorilla brain for once in a way, and the baboon brain also under the fancy of their being *degraded* forms" (his emphasis, *Life and Works* 3: 148). As Kingsley ceaselessly reminds the young reader of *Water Babies*, "your soul makes your body"; those boys who do not, through the quest, make themselves as imperial men, degenerate into efts, and the Do-As-You-Likes turn into apes like Rolleston's gorilla. Nation is created through the quest, and the quest can only be fulfilled through and by the clean and proper white body of the benevolent male imperialist, who vampirically channels the primitive vigor of the feminine other through his own body, draining her of her racial difference. Cholera is the marker of the inappropriately needy, dependent, open male body, racialized through this dependence—a marker of the sin of enslavement and exploitation. The goal of empire—perfect health and whiteness for all—will mark both the fulfillment of nation and the culmination of individual spiritual development.

CONCLUSION

> In a family as long descended as the Walters, there are bound to be a few carried off by plague. . . . Black Jack. Came from a water pump, half the city of London, can you imagine? (93)

> The worst thing about being sick in America, Ethel, is you are booted out of the parade. Americans have no use for sick. (210)

> —Tony Kushner, *Angels in America*

The cholera qua cholera played a relatively small role in the literature of the day, although the roles of "fever," which coded cholera and other poverty-related diseases, and of the sanitary movement were vast. What is clear in its fitful appearances in propria persona, however, is its enduring connection to a particular conception of poverty—as the result of inadequacies in the social sphere—and the connection of that social insufficiency to a racialized body that is inadequately independent. In nonliterary discourse, the presence of cholera was as pervasive as it was symbolically overdetermined. Cholera's presence or absence was made to index governmental irresponsibility, national sinfulness, the immorality or oppression of the poor worker, and the modernity or barbarism of the metropole and its colonies. The body and its health became the basic unit of measurement for the success of the social body and the modernity of the nation. This was made possible by a rich complex of scientific, medical, and social theories that grounded national cultural identity ever more insistently in the raced, classed, gendered body. By the mid-Victorian period, discourses on health, especially public health, permeated the very idea of civilization, of nation, and of the state. They continue to do so today.

Eugenic theories of public health lost credence dramatically after the horrifying excesses of World War II, which drove European and U.S. rhetorics of national identity based on race and hygiene from the public sphere. Still, notions of intrinsic dirtiness and disease continue to shape the West's response to "developing" countries, replication nineteenth-century colonial relations in twenty-first-century global dynamics. Although Western nations have largely ceased to make overtly racist claims about the superiority of certain kinds of bodies and locations, the Western response to ongoing health crises in Africa, Eastern Europe, the Caribbean, and portions of Asia—a confused mixture of genuine concern, blaming the victims, trade and immigration cordon sanitaires, and ineffectual paternalism—reflect a pattern of continued self-construction based on ideals of health, cleanliness, and modernity that often do not reflect real conditions. (For example, U.S. maternal mortality, a chief index of public health effectiveness, is comparable to that of Slovenia and Hungary, and is substantially worse than most Western European countries, and such other countries as Kuwait and Croatia. However, in the U.S. imagination, these countries are often thought of as backward and disease-prone compared to the United States.⁹ Similarly, continuing construction today of AIDS and other diseases as "African" or "Asian" diseases follows a familiar pattern, as did early 1980s construction of AIDS as a "sin" disease in the United States caused by homosexuality and drug addiction. Like cholera, AIDS was read as a disease of the weak and intemperate in the West and as a disease endemic to nonwhite communities, who exacerbated it with their immoral behavior.

This is, of course, an old pattern—one might think of the construction of leprosy in the Middle Ages as a Jewish disease spreading in the European population through lechery. However, the epidemic disease's fundamental importance to the rhetoric of nation is a modern phenomenon. Its importance is recognized now, as it was in the nineteenth century, by authors and activists, who respond to its now tactfully submerged, but continuing presence. The U.S. response provides an excellent—one might say paradigmatic—example of the response of the modern Western imperial power to AIDS. Tony Kushner's *Angels in America*, written in the early 1990s but set in the 1980s period of the early epidemic and then-President Ronald Reagan's response, drama-tizes the rhetoric of health and morality that still lies at the basis of nation in the United States.

The response of conservative evangelicals to AIDS in 1980s America is well documented. Jerry Falwell thundered, "AIDS is the wrath of God upon homosexuals," and Reagan's communications director Pat Buchanan opined that AIDS is "nature's revenge on gay men." Early reporting on the origin of the disease targeted Africa and African diasporic communities, such as black Haitians. Kushner's rhetoric of millennialism and multiculturalism, his char-acterization of America as a "melting pot where nothing ever melted" (16), of an absent God and panicked angels milling around like incompetent middle managers left running a failing business by an irresponsible CEO, echoes and inverts reactionary coverage of the AIDS crisis in the early years. His val-orization of difference—sexual, racial, national—as a source of redemption rather than of disease and death is a direct response to the paranoia of the dis-course around the epidemic. And his play recognizes that, as is often the case when disease becomes a public event, what is at stake in these discourses is a notion of identity, especially national identity. This identity is based in the ideal of the white, heterosexual, American male who finally cannot be found in the play, because he does not exist.

The imperial lineage of America as white nation tends toward sterility for Kushner. Prior Walter, the man ill with AIDS who is the principal pro-tagonist of the play, traces his roots to England. His family came over on the Mayflower—but Kushner reminds us that even the Englishness of England is vexed as the Walters came to England with the Norman invaders of 1066. Prior sees visions of his ancestors interspersed with visits from the angel who wishes him, as a reverse messiah, to end the messiness of the failed world, infected with the "virus of time" and history. Kushner explicitly links AIDS to cholera and the black plague, as the two ghosts who appear to Prior explain that they have died of those epidemics; in his way the political entail-ments of epidemics are emphasized as part of a continuing and specifically European narrative.

But Prior chooses life, with all its embodied messiness, disease, suffering, and human connection; he chooses against the impossible sterility valorized by villain Roy Cohn, who dies of AIDS hanging on to his racism and racist desire, his self-loathing homophobia and anti-Semitism, the dark side of the aesthetics of the idealized body as nation. If Falwell echoes sermons of 1832, then Kushner's insistence on the relation between AIDS rhetoric, homopho-bia, and the history of capitalist oppression (Cohn is haunted by the ghost of Ethel Rosenberg), recalls shades of Henry Hetherington. In the effort to reclaim and valorize the diseased body as formative of a discourse of nation, Kushner rewrites the literary tradition presented in Eliot and Kingsley. If

Cohn represents the conservative vision of the nation as body—"Americans have no use of sick" (210)—the black nurse Belize states the case for the opposite view, that America is itself a sick body: "Terminal, crazy and mean" (233). But the rabbi who opens the trilogy with a eulogy for an anonymous immigrant woman has it right when he reminds us that these are all constructions having a tenuous relation to reality: "You do not live in America. No such place exists" (16).

Like nation, the ideal and invulnerable body is a myth, one that easily becomes a pernicious fetish. When this body becomes central to nation itself, it can create a dangerous logic of judgment and exclusion, as both this volume and studies of fascist body aesthetics in the early twentieth century have abundantly illustrated. Within the liberal paradigm, it contributed to pathologize the political views and values of nonwhites, of women, and of the poor, allowing the illusion if inclusion, without the reality. But it also can (and did) create an emphasis on public health and universal education that eventually created hitherto unparalleled opportunities for civic culture that in turn allowed for a more inclusive model of the social body. In short, as the body came to be the very site of the articulation of identity and representation within politics, wielded by elites, it could also be used as a powerful site of resistance by the oppressed. As the ideal body became the measure of nation, the stunted bodies of factory children reproached the wealthy. In the twentieth century, the inversion of a dominant bodily aesthetic ("Black is beautiful!) was a rallying cry that encompassed more abstract legal and political issues. This volume has attempted to trace a small but significant part of the history of this complex becoming.

NOTES

INTRODUCTION

1. See for example "An Account of the Disease Termed Cholera Morbus, from Its First Appearance at Sunderland, to Its Final Departure from Northumberland and Durham, with the Daily Official Reports of Its Destructive Ravages in Newcastle and Gateshead." Many accounts, including this one, include a narrative of the Great Plague of 1636. See also Henry Gaulter, *The Origin and Progress of the Malignant Cholera in Manchester*.

2. Dhiman Barua and William B. Greenough, writing in 1992, observe that death may occur within a few hours and often within the first twenty-four, with an untreated death rate of up to seventy percent (217), though most other sources list fifty percent as standard. They observe that the average fluid loss for a 40 kilometer (about 88 pounds) Bengali male is 25 to 30 liters (roughly 5.5 to 8 gallons), but loss of up to 80 liters (over 21 gallons) has been documented (this last, obviously is only possible with continuous fluid replacement).

3. Secondary symptoms included, according to Goodeve, uraemia, cholera typhoid, ulceration of the cornea (especially in India), gangrene of penis, scrotum, and mucous membrane of the mouth. Also occasionally present were gangrenous tip of the nose, swelling of parotid glands, bedsores, and lung inflammation. Gregory also refers to a tendency to develop lung inflammation in the second, feverish stage in some patients (1846, 642). Today, Barua and Greenough list the following as the possible complications following cholera, usually due to prolonged shock: "pneumonia"—which was probably a large contributor to what nineteenth-century medics thought of as the "typhoid" phase—"sepsis, renal failure, hypoglycemia, corneal ulceration, electrolyte abnormalities, and cardiac abnormalities" (218).

4. I use the term "medics," following historian Frank Mort, to include the whole panoply of medical practitioners in Victorian England. Later, I discuss the range of medical professionals operating in this period.

5. See especially Rosenberg for a historical discussion of cholera in the United States; Durey and Morris for Britain; Bourdelais, Kudlick or Delaporte for France; McGrew for Russia; and Evans's marvelous *Death in Hamburg* for Germany.

6. Cholera is still an important epidemic disease today in Africa, India, and Latin America, and is considered endemic in many other parts of the world, including the Gulf coast of the United States. What Barua and Greenough define as the "seventh pandemic" began in 1961 and is still ongoing at the time of this writing (16–17).

7. A word is in order here about the use of the term "liberal," which I use not in the specific sense of the Liberal party (except when capitalized) or of a very particular political theory. There were many kinds of liberals, of course, in mid-Victorian society, espousing political theories from the economic liberalism of Smith to that of the later Mill, which emphasized social responsibility while retaining a largely Kantian notion of a core individual self. But I am referring here to the overarching philosophy of government in the period stemming from Enlightenment ideals and largely shared by Tory and Whig, and later by Conservative, Liberal, and most Radicals alike. These ideals include the conviction that government should in some sense be representative, should interest itself in building the good society (or on removing impediments to its development), should be based when feasible on consent rather than force, and should be founded on the inviolability of property and a relatively free circulation of labor, capital, and goods. It is, then, at base, a capitalist and possessive individualist vision. There were many different takes on what each of these core terms meant, but this was basically the ideal of government that most Victorians shared, and that comes under the broad term "liberal." Thus, many people identified economic and social policies as "liberal," especially in the beginning of the period, that we would see as very conservative today because they were based on a fundamentalist view of economic liberalism. By the time the Liberal party came along, the term had become more clearly associated with social policies favoring the extension of the franchise and later, institutional social measures such as universal education. But I am using the term here in its most catholic sense, and in that sense, Victorian Britain was marked by a steadily liberalizing vision of government.

8. See Thomas Richards's *The Imperial Archive* for a thorough discussion of the status of the archive.

9. The most famous of these statements is Margaret Pelling's: "All the known epidemic diseases were exceeded in incidence and effect by the many forms of tuberculosis. . . . Cholera has, however, attracted some of the kind of attention from historians that other diseases, excepting plague, have conspicuously lacked" (*Cholera, Fever, and English Medicine* 4). Typhus and typhoid and other endemics killed many more than cholera. Still, although its epidemiological importance might have been overstressed by historians, present-day scholars could hardly emphasize its *social* importance more than did the Victorians themselves.

CHAPTER 1. A SINFUL NATION: 1832

1. Rosenberg, who insightfully discusses the contradictions between the theological and scientific arguments, comes to the surprising conclusion that the two domains were so socially segregated as not to create significant conflict, as early as the '30s. This is incorrect. The conflict was both significant and unresolved until the mid '50s (114).

2. Obviously, I am homogenizing two groups here that have broad interests in common. Within these groups are many factions and individuals with different views and agendas that I cannot explore here, but which are certainly worth pursuing.

3. I am using "Britain" here loosely. The authors I cite use the term "nation" in a slippery and loose sense, depending largely on context and rhetorical purpose. Sometimes they are referring to Britain, and sometimes to England. The Anglican Church, of course, was not the established church of Scotland, though it was, at this point, of England, Ireland, and Wales.

4. J. C. D. Clark, *English Society: 1688–1832*, provides an extensive analysis of the political and ideological centrality of the Anglican church-state connection in these three legislative actions. Popular reform agitation after the first defeat of the bill was particularly anticlerical.

5. Eileen Groth Lyon identifies a trend in conservative churchmen's writings about the "contagion" of infidelity as early as 1810 (55).

6. That is, tenants or owners of property valued, at a minimum, at £10 per year.

7. For a detailed study of the geography of religious affiliation, see B. I. Coleman, *The Church of England.*

8. Margot Finn, in *After Chartism*, cites examples of sermons appealing to the concept of nation as early as the early seventeenth century (38–39).

9. Yet, it is important to note that repeal of the Test and Corporations Acts was generally supported by the episcopate (Brose 15). Anti-reformers were not a fully unified group, but a very vocal minority that overlapped with church leaders on some issues and not on others.

10. Although the sermon literature on national sin was most fully developed during the first two cholera epidemics, two later events drew a significant body of publications in this area, both associated with their own fast days. The first, during the Crimean War, didn't generally expend much time on defining nation. The sense of sin was vague and people were largely exhorted to look to their own sins. (An exception was John Alcock, an Anglican obviously feeling embattled in Dublin, who took a historical approach, tying toleration of Indian religion to toleration of Catholicism. His text refers back to 1829 and the traumatic removal of Catholic Disabilities, connecting it to the cholera of 1832, the mid-century cholera, and cattle plague, and so on until the occasion of his own sermon in 1855.) The second, associated with the Sepoy uprising of 1857, was more extensive, and tended to dwell on the national sin of not encouraging or forcing Christianity upon the natives. Occasionally, other specific issues were named: for example, Thomas Snead Hughes mentioned the English role in forcing the opium trade upon the Chinese. A vocal minority directed attention to England's (or Britain's) abuse of India—Edmund Kell's sermon on the subject went through at least four editions and garnered enough critical attention to inspire him to publish a response to a reviewer in pamphlet form. Many sermons on this topic called for revenge, and a few for forgiveness, that the minority who did seriously engage issues of national identity tended to do so in terms of Christianity (Protestant, usually Anglican) versus native religions.

11. Interestingly enough, however, in France, where Catholicism was the majority religion, Catholic clergy cited cholera as God's vengeance on the French for their irreligious attitudes and failure to support the Bourbons, attempting to use the cholera to renew its authority (Delaporte 60).

12. Edward Bouverie Pusey, close friend of Keble and Newman, was strongly associated with the Tractarian movement and the Catholic revival, though he never converted, as Newman did. Such movements, emphasizing ritual and episcopal authority, were seen by many Anglicans as moving suspiciously close to Catholicism.

13. This distinction clearly emerged from some well-defined point of dissemination and was widely repeated—perhaps it came from an ex cathedra or pastoral communication that I have not been able to find. Almost the exact same language is used in John Alcock's "National Sins and National Calamity. A Sermon preached in Bethesda Chapel, Dublin, Wed., March 21, 1855" (the day of prayer and fasting for the Crimean War). And again in Reverend J. Leech Porter's [curate of Shipley-cum-Heaton] "Nations are punished and rewarded *now*, but individuals *hereafter*. . . . Nations have no further existence in their *national* capacity—as collective bodies their being is not perpetuated beyond the boundaries of time, and so they exist not *as nations* to be judged in eternity for national sins" (11–12).

14. As we still do today. The 1990s' outbreak of what was called "Asian flu" when overextended Southeast Asian markets crashed and their currency devalued was handled in the U.S. press in terms of infection and containment.

CHAPTER 2. AFTER 1832: MEDICAL AUTHORITY AND THE CLERGY

1. Curiously, in all four epidemics, there were almost no references by the Anglican clergy to the many other countries suffering simultaneously during the pandemics. The nation, it appears, had to be defined separately from a global identity.

2. As Benedict Anderson has argued.

3. The history of contagionism and anti-contagionism is complex as each of these "positions" actually embraced many medical theories within it. However, in broad terms, we can define these here as the positions supporting direct human spread of the cholera versus those who believed epidemics were spread by some other means, perhaps climatic. Sanitarians, as believing that disease was caused by filth rather than contact with the sick, fell largely, if problematically, into the anti-contagionist camp. Although anti-contagionism was arguably the dominant medical paradigm in the 1830s, a stance that, not incidentally, supported commercial interests that would have been damaged by quarantines, it required constant defense against a popular common sense that "the Fever" (a large category of disease under which cholera was often subsumed by medics and laypeople alike) was contagious.

4. Palmerston was home secretary when he wrote this letter; he was to become prime minister in 1854.

5. For more on the representation of hidden urban depths in this period, especially in reference to the work of John Snow, see my *Mapping the Victorian Social Body* (2004).

6. The parish's name is sometimes spelled St. James and other times St. James's. I have followed the more popular style of calling it St. James's, except in titles and direct quotes where the spelling differs.

7. See, for example, Cyrus Edson.

8. See Phillip A. Nicholls.

9. As Anne Digby, Jeanne Peterson, and Irvine Loudon have all discussed.

10. John Henry Newman was one of the principal authors of the *Tracts for the Times*, which launched the Tractarian movement, with which he was identified until his conversion to Roman Catholicism in 1845. In the tracts, Newman argued for Episcopal authority in the Church of England based on direct apostolic succession.

11. James Glaisher (1809–1903) is best known as a meteorologist, but also maintained a lively interest in sanitary theory. Cholera, like many epidemic diseases, was often believed to be caused by bad air and wind conditions, and it was conventional to include meteorological information in sanitary reports. Glaisher here reports on a blue mist supposed to be associated with the presence of the cholera.

12. This liturgy was slightly modified in 1866 in order to take into account the rinderpest, or cattle plague, another national calamity "running" simultaneously with cholera.

13. See Michel Foucault, "Governmentality" and Poovey, *Making a Social Body*.

CHAPTER 3. A SUFFERING NATION:
RESPONSES OF THE POOR AND RADICALS TO THE CHOLERA

1. I use the masculine pronoun deliberately; the expansion of suffrage was limited to males.

2. For discussions of the perception of the body as problematic by nature of its physicality and also as identified with the social body, cf. Catherine Gallagher and Mary Poovey. For the treatment of the poor as a passive "aggregate body," see Poovey, 78–88.

3. In an 1848 letter to the *Times* editor, the anonymous writer asserts, "It was well known that many of the inhabitants of the parish denied the fact that cholera prevailed at that time [1832] in the metropolis" ("Cholera in Whitechapel").

4. The best coverage of the social response is still Morris, *Cholera 1832*.

5. As Durey notes, on at least one occasion a purely rhetorical offering of a feast day was misunderstood, leaving thousands of poor stranded, having expected to be fed (198).

6. This fast is a response to famine, not the cholera.

7. It is extremely unlikely that any medic was paid at this rate.

8. This combination of explanations that were elsewhere explicitly opposed to each other (sanitarian explanations that were generally anticontagionist and contagionist theories) is actually coherent with later "contingent contagionist" theories that held that cholera was not normally contagious but could become so under certain conditions. Here, however, it is probably simply too early for these two positions to have hardened into an opposition that would have required explanation. It is likely that this writer sees no contradiction between the two models.

9. For more discussions, see Durey, Morris, and Shapter.

10. Durey lists this man as "Hare," but the original newspaper sources say Hase (180).

11. Durey attributes much of the anti-cholera violence to its unfortunate concurrence with the Anatomy Act.

12. See Richardson and Durey for extended discussions of such practices.

13. The upper classes were not immune from the same fears, as this August 11, 1866, letter in the *Press and St. James Chronicle* illustrates: "It is almost impossible to contain one's indignation when reading of the matter-of-course way in which cholera patients are made to propagate the disease by the aid of street cabs. At the Thames Police Court, under the eyes . . . of the magistrate himself, we find a patient in an advanced state of cholera removed in a cab. . . . It seems awful to contemplate that we are liable, on hailing a cab, to occupy a seat which has just been vacated by a patient in the last stage of Asiatic cholera" ("The Cholera" 508).

14. The letters to the Commissioners of Sewers are housed in the Guildhall archives.

15. As noted in 1849, "Plunder of Cholera Patients," which also refers to resistance to removal of the bodies.

16. Tract writer Mrs. Carleton, advancing her hydrogen theory of cholera, opines, "Influenza is a relation of the Cholera—a noble relation, uncontaminated by earthly emanations, a polite kind of cholera for the aristocracy, that keeps aloof from noxious exhalations, produced, perhaps, by minor currents of hydrogen proceeding in advance of the great choleraic current" (54). Although Mrs. Carleton is hardly an example of mainstream medical theory, she does provide an illustration of a pervasive popular attitude that cholera was not a "polite" disease, nor should respectable people be vulnerable to it.

CHAPTER 4. MEDICS AND THE PUBLIC SPHERE

1. Amazingly, by the 1860s, even the abdomen was routinely entered due to obstetric contributions to knowledge (Lawrence 26).

2. See Lindsay Granshaw (232).

3. See Loudon for an extended discussion.

4. As John Pickstone puts it, in Kay-Shuttleworth's text, "The mass of the poor lay effectively unconnected to the centres of consciousness; thus the tendency to corruption went unchecked. . . . The poor were de-moralized, by subtraction merely carnal; left alone, the physical passions were destructive. The answer, of course, was moral education" (Pickstone 413–14).

5. As Nicholas Coles has observed, Kay-Shuttleworth conflates the poor with their disease and their disease with their habitation, then anthropomorphizes those habitations as a malicious and sexualized threat (73).

6. However, Chadwick had no hesitation in using the public support he mobilized for public health measures for his own directly political aims. The water companies ran afoul of Chadwick and other sanitarians when they failed to be adequately responsive to public need during the cholera of 1848–1849, allowing "public outrage [to become] . . . organized political activity through the efforts of engineers, speculators and sanitarians" (Hamlin, *A Science* 100–01) who had various stakes in seeing the control of the companies challenged, even though no real change took place until after the epidemic of 1866 (Hamlin, *A Science* 104). The tradition of using the public health office as a bully pulpit continued after Chadwick's departure. Hamlin points out that by 1867 Frankland and other public officials were consciously choosing, as a matter of policy, to present health information (about water purity, in this case) in an inflammatory and exaggerated manner to the public, in order to effect change (*A Science* 161).

7. See Roy Lewis and Angus Maude; see also Anne Witz.

8. Anne Digby has pointed out that the 1858 Act did not achieve closure for all medics either (31), but it was a good beginning.

9. Women's professional organizations tended to come to closure later, lacking access to the civil and institutional mechanisms that enabled it. Further, women's professions, because they *were* women's, tended to be labeled semi-professions (Witz 60–61).

10. Mary Poovey and Jacques Donzelot place the earliest elaboration of the social in the late eighteenth century; others, such as Patrick Joyce and Nikolas Rose, have argued that the nineteenth century is largely a period before the social—certainly, if one defines the social as T. H. Marshall does, in terms of rights, this is true. But for my purposes here, I will be defining it as a broader cultural phenomenon.

11. Jane Lewis has observed that "Social policies were only becoming matters of 'high politics' in the period 1870–1914" (3). This is indeed the case because until the 1860s the social had not yet so visibly permeated all areas of economic and political life as to require institutionalization, which would serve to paradoxically strip it of a certain kind of authority derived from its separation from the political and economic, while at the same time legitimating its power—and to some extent that of feminism in this period—by institutionally validating the centrality of the social to the formation of the modern state.

12. See Gilbert, *The Citizen's Body*, for a discussion of the relation of the social to the public and private.

13. John Snow and William Budd, Hamlin notes, were outside the sanitary establishment (*Public Health* 244).

14. For more on this, see Radhika Ramasubban.

15. See John Eyler for an excellent discussion of Farr's attitudes and their development over time.

16. See *Parliamentary Papers* XIX (1842): 93–122.

17. The standard nosology used until then, William Cullen's, "had been ruled by a primary emphasis on function, both on the general and on the local level; Farr referred all local conditions, which included the greater number of diseased states, to a site" (Pelling 94), but stayed away from limiting disease species to the requirement of self-reproduction (Pelling 95).

18. Farr also, like the sanitarians, who were strongly Benthamite, connected his medical project with political economy. In the tradition of Adam Smith, Farr regarded a man's earning capacity as his value and represented public health in financial terms (Eyler 92–96).

19. For an explicit reference to incest, for example, see Chadwick, 193.

20. The following fanciful introduction to a *City Press* article on local government provides an excellent example of a deliberate use of a trope that had become, for many, an unconscious way of envisioning the city: "The best performance in the fantoccini is that of the figure which, in the act of dancing, becomes disjointed yet every joint, still pregnant with vitality, continues to dance as gaily as ever. . . . So long as the machinery is perfect, and the performer sober, all goes well; but if the main string should break, the figure would fall in a disjointed wreck. . . . The metropolis is very like that figure. When we first view it as a whole, it appears to be complete and closely knit, and its actions are energetic if not graceful. If we continue to observe we see in due time that its several limbs or component parts are easily separated, that after separation they are still vital and active, generally speaking more active than before, and so the dance goes on quite gaily. But if the string should break that ties the whole together! Awful thought, that a social chaos must be the consequence . . . it is worn to a thread, it does not act its part with integrity, and here and there a limb separated from the rest, and, energetically kicking, refuses to glide back to its place in the metropolitan anatomy. If we could get the figure to stand still for a moment, we should behold it in its perfection, but, unhappily, it is full of life, and that, so to speak, is death for it, for the limbs will get away from the trunk" ("Metropolitan Confusions" 4).

21. The emphasis on the skin in this excerpt, and on the Ladies' Sanitary Association tract quoted before it, is characteristic of this period, as I shall discuss in chapter 5.

22. My point here is not that this is the first or only time this had ever happened, but it is probably the first time that conditions were ripe for medics to take advantage of that public presence and establish themselves as a profession whose interests were appropriately public, not as well-educated individuals but as medics.

CHAPTER 5. THE BODY IN QUESTION

1. William Baly and William W. Gull's *Reports on the Epidemic Cholera. Drawn up at the Desire of the Cholera Committee of the Royal College of Physicians*, provides an excellent overview of the six then-current theories (4–5), enumerated below.

1. The General Board of Health theorized, "that the disease spreads by an 'atmospheric influence or epidemic constitution,' its progress consisting of a succession of local outbreaks, and that the particular localities affected are determined by certain 'localizing conditions,' which are, first, all those well-known circumstances which render places insalubrious; and, second, a susceptibility of the disease in the inhabitants of such places, produced by the habitual respiration of an impure atmosphere" (4).
2. Many medics believed that "following the analogy of diseases known to be due to morbid poisons regards the cause of Cholera as a morbific matter which undergoes increase only within the human body, and is propagated by means of emanations from the bodies of the sick, in other words, by contagion" (4). In a footnote, they explain that the term "infection" will only be used in the most general sense of "pollution" in this report.
3. Snow argued that the disease was waterborne (5).
4. Other medics believed "that the cause . . . is a morbific matter or poison, but supposes that it is reproduced only in the air, not within the bodies of those whom it affects, and that its diffusion is due to the agency of the atmosphere" (5).
5. Another theory "admits that the cholera matter is increased by a species of fermentation or other mode of reproduction in impure, damp, and stagnant air, but maintains that it nevertheless is distributed and diffused by means of human intercourse; it being carried in ships and other vehicles, and even in the clothes of men, especially the foul clothes of vagrants, and the accumulated baggage of armies" (5).
6. The last theory "combines the second and the fourth, assuming that the material causes of the disease may be increased and propagated in and by impure air, as well as in and by the human body" (5).

Baly and Gull conclude that states of air are very important, as are topography, population density, and sewerage. Baly and Gull are both anti-contagionist and anti-Snow.

2. George Gregory notes that he saw nurses in St. Giles "fall successively victims to the disease" (1846, 533).

3. Arthur Sansom in his 1866 tract on cholera dismisses "cholera mist"—heavy blue mist that hangs over an affected area and refuses to blow away—as an urban legend. John Chapman, however, documents cholera mist as a fact in his medical textbook of the same year (ix).

4. One anonymous author argued in the *Times* that "[discharges] are comparatively non-infectious at the moment when they are discharged, but afterwards, while undergoing decomposition, acquire their *maximum* of infectious power" ("Precautions Against Cholera").

5. As Hamlin points out, "monocausal" explanations for epidemics were not well received by medics in an intellectual climate that favored multicausal explanations for disease (*A Science* 113).

6. "Bleeding is often necessary with this stimulation because the action of the heart is so weak that it does not keep up enough of motion in the blood to prevent it from coagulating, and unless the freedom of circulations be assisted by venesection, the stimulants cannot give the heart power enough; and though the blood may have begun to thicken and 'oozes out at first like treacle,' the renewed motion as it flows makes it fluid" (122).

7. "Previous to the visitation of cholera in 1831, before I had an opportunity of personal observation, I was led (by reading letters from India, and books) to make a too-limited estimate of the other symptoms of cholera, referring chiefly to the affection of the stomach and bowels. . . . When, however, I encountered the enemy hand to hand, I saw at once that it was a febrile disease. . . . This is already granted by some; to others . . . it may seem a startling assertion . . . proper remedies [are] . . . fever remedies," but stimulants are hurtful (Billing 249–50).

8. John Syer Bristow (1827–1895), physician and pathology expert, attended at St. Thomas's Hospital 1849–1892.

9. Durey asserts that bleeding fell out of favor after 1832 (124–25), but in my reading of case notes, I found that it had wide currency much later.

10. Billing (1791–1881) studied originally in Dublin and attended for many years at the London Hospital. He became an examiner in medicine at the University of London and published six editions of his popular textbook. He also wrote a treatise on cholera in 1848. He specialized in diseases of the chest.

11. Billing writes, "The *modes* by which students may attain a *knowledge* of the *nature* of *disease*, after learning physiology or the nature of healthy functions (which is obtainable in lectures), are, accurate observation of the diseases which take place in external parts as they are submitted to our senses in CLINICAL SURGERY, and in the functions of internal parts as met with in CLINICAL MEDICINE; and MORBID ANATOMY, the examination of of [sic] what is the degree and nature of the alteration which has taken place in the structure which is the seat of the disease" (Billing's emphasis, 1831, 1–2).

12. George Gregory (1790–1853) studied physic in Edinburgh and later became M.R.C.S. in England, and did duty as a military surgeon. He was a specialist in fevers.

13. The four new areas are: 1. Sources of disease with new material on morbid poison, miasma and contagion, two new diseases: "Cow Pox and malignant Cholera" (Gregory vi), and several new phenomena "which exist within the frame itself"; 2. Detection of disease; 3. Seats of disease; 4. Effects of disease (morbid anatomy).

14. Cholera, interestingly, is under chronic diseases of the viscera, so that "acute" does not have the same force that we might expect, and that suggests a response to the postmortem findings of irritated bowels in cholera patients. He sees it simply as the worst form of diarrheal disease, although he also acknowledges its epidemic character.

15. James Russell Reynolds (1828–1896) was a renowned physician and expert on nervous disorders, who was particularly interested in clinical uses of electricity. He taught at the University College of London, and was for some time the president of the Royal College of Physicians. He was created a baronet in 1895.

16. Still, he retains the typical mid-century distinction in the book's organization: "It is proposed to make the first division of diseases into their two great groups— 1st, those in which the whole organism appears primarily and prominently deranged [like influenza], and 2nd, those in which special organs or systems of organs, are, in like manner, affected. Subdividing the first group we have two classes; A, those in which the disease appears to be caused [by outside influences] . . . and B, those in which the malady seems to depend on some internal change . . . [the second group is subdivided by organ systems] that systems of organs, are, in like manner, affected" (1866, 24–25).

17. Galen was a second-century Greek medic, whose theories that the body was composed of four fluids, or humors (blood, yellow and black bile, and phlegm), that all had to be in balance continued to be influential well into the nineteenth century, persisting at the popular level long after they were discarded by professional medics.

18. See Thomas Laqueur's *Making Sex*, for example.

19. Erin O'Connor has argued that there are racial anxieties associated with this blackening of the body by an invasive colonial disease as well.

20. See, for example, George Gregory, who notes unusual muscular contractions after death he believes are specific to cholera (532).

21. Thomas Mann's *Death in Venice*, in 1912, mentions cholera sicca: "the 'dry' type, the most malignant form of the contagion. In this form, the victim's body loses the power to expel the water secreted by the blood vessels, it shrivels up, he passes with hoarse cries from convulsion to convulsion, his blood grows thick like pitch, and he suffocates in a few hours" (64). The dry disease can also simply take the form of unconsciousness before a speedy death, as it does with his protagonist, Aschenbach. Mann also describes "intemperance, indecency and increase of crime" as well as "professional vice" and murder under cover of the plague (65).

22. Erin O'Connor details the racialization of cholera corpses in her recent book *Raw Material*.

CHAPTER 6. RACE, GENDER, AND CHOLERA

1. It is also possible that the loss of British troops in India to cholera during and following the mutiny—most dramatically exemplified in Havelock's losses, which delayed the arrival of troops in Kanpur—identified cholera in the eyes of the British public with Indian hostility to British rule. Many writers of the time describe the epidemic as being as if the land itself conspired against them.

2. See, for example, David Arnold's analysis of the association of effeminacy with the tropics, especially as applied to Bengal in *The Problem of Nature*.

3. See Pamela Gilbert, *Mapping the Victorian Social Body*, for a full discussion.

4. See Mark Harrison, *Public Health*, for a discussion of this point of view.

5. De Renzy went on to quarrel with Cuningham, the Surgeon General of India, because de Renzy supported Snow's theory against the anti-contagionist doctrines of Cuningham (Hume 712).

6. There were two dominant Indian medical systems: ayurvedic medicine practiced by Hindu health-care providers called *vaids* (or *vaidyas*), and *unani*, practiced by Muslim *hakims*. By mid-century, British medics distrusted these local medical providers, but also objected to the use of British-trained Indian and Eurasian doctors in public medicine (Harrison 32–34). In this way they both guaranteed a stranglehold on public health, and, indeed, strangled it—for lack of human resources. In fact, colonial public medicine was very important to the British, in part for the information that it provided about that population, in statistical form (Arnold, *Imperial Medicine* 17).

7. Harrison charts the admiration of Surgeon Sir Whitelaw Ainslie and others, who, in the 1820s, studied Indian indigenous medicine and found much to respect in it. Yet, by the mid-century, local practitioners were distrusted by the British as quacks who retarded the progress of scientific medicine (Harrison, *Public Health in British India* 16, 41, 53). Harrison attributes some of this change to the rebellion/mutiny and some to the changes in European medicine from a humoral system more closely resembling Indian schemas to the scientific medical model. Arnold, however locates the shift earlier, in 1835, and notes that it was not so much a significant change in attitude as the further manifestation of an existing tendency to privilege Western medicine while taking what was useful from native traditions (*Colonizing the Body*, see chapter 2).

8. See also Klein, "Death in India."

9. See also Klein, "Cholera, Dysentery and Development."

10. For example the zamindari system of land ownership engineered by the British encouraged what Klein calls a "crazy quilt of irrigation" systems that caused the degradation of natural waterways in Bengal and their ability to cleanse themselves ("Imperialism" 512).

11. Watts's book is a lively, although highly partisan and occasionally inaccurate synthesis of the existing research.

12. The British colonial government viewed the propitiatory activities of natives regarding these deities, sometimes involving parades and *devis* (women dressed up as the goddess, and sometimes believed to be possessed by her), with disgust and alarm (Arnold, "Cholera" 132)—despite the fact that Britain's first response had been religious observances and propitiatory activities also. (I haven't come across any nineteenth-century Britons who observed the irony.) British officials noted the Indians' connection of cholera with British rule, so that religious anti-cholera activities were suspected of political meanings and watched carefully (Arnold, "Cholera" 134). Further, Indians' reaction to Western medicine was equivocal. David Arnold has argued that, although Indians sometimes welcomed British medicine and used it side by side with other modes of treatment, some Indians also felt upset by such practices. Because

of British medicine's emphasis on dissection, and Hindu repulsion for such intimate handling of unclean materials, as well as for the notion of dissection itself, "Western medicine itself bore the taint, the stigma, of the pariah, . . . that seemed to situate its practitioners among the outcaste and defiled" (Arnold, *Colonizing the Body* 5).

13. Prashad times this perception in 1832; in fact, at least in Britain, the dramatic racialization of the disease doesn't begin until the '60s. More typical in the '30s were arguments that Indian and English cholera were not the same disease and that there was nothing to be gained by perusing Indian reports. But, as Prashad himself and others have pointed out, early observers' praise for or wonder at the constant bathing practices of Indians gave way to descriptions of their filthy practices that contaminated the water. Rather than being credited with a desire for cleanliness, by mid-century, Indian bathing practices were described as purely motivated by superstition, and like all their superstitious (that is, religious) practices, productive of disease.

14. All things Eastern were suspect, and cholera represented the *ne plus ultra* of all evil things Eastern. In his biographical memoir on John Snow, Richardson cites an occasion wherein at a lecture, Snow was asked, "as a poser," where the first cholera cell had come from. He answered, "tell me where the first tiger or the first upas tree came from, nay, tell me where you came from yourself" (quoted in Snow, *Snow on Cholera* xlv). Obviously, Snow is using "tiger" or "upas tree" to some extent at random, but the immediate association shows the degree to which the disease evoked negative representations of the Far East, and of course, Snow had studied the Indian documents at length. He also apparently grew fond of this comparison; this same example pops up in Snow's essay "On Continuous Molecular Changes" (*Snow on Cholera* 171). As Prashad writes: "India (they) acts as a metaphor for all that the European (we) is not. What *they* are, fits for *them*, since it is the natural environment which *they* need 'in order to prosper.' [For 'them'] The filth is not filth" (256). This attitude made it possible to leave Indians in the Augean stables that imperialism had helped create, but that, in the perception of many British, was an unalterable part of the landscape. As we have seen, however, Indians did *not* prosper in this environment.

15. Ironically, British deforestation and irrigation created breeding grounds for mosquitoes and literally made the environment more "tropical" in the negative sense the term had acquired for Europeans, which then justified domination of Indians who were believed to be the racially degenerate products of such an environment. As Arnold points out, although India never became a "neo-Europe," the European impact on the land and people was nonetheless profound (*Problem* 176). Britain exploited what was specifically non-European about the Indian environment, for example, to grow crops like tea and cotton that would not grow in Europe, aggressively assimilating India's image (and sometimes its actual geography) to those "tropical" purposes.

16. See Antoinette Burton's *Burdens of History* for an excellent discussion of British women's views of Indian gender relations.

17. One might think that British medics at home would have placed a premium on the advice of medics experienced with the cholera in India. In fact, there was relatively little "crossover" between their work until the mid-century, when the massive influx of troops after the rebellion and the expansion of the profession made what

would be called "tropical medicine" an emerging field. Although many medics working in India published in Britain during the early 1830s, in letters to the *Lancet* and the like, many, if not most British medics in Britain dismissed their advice, suggesting that cholera on European terrain and in a European population at home was a very different disease process than it was in any population in India. Although this attitude was consonant with beliefs about disease at the time, it may also have been influenced by an attitude among domestic medics ranging from patronizing to contemptuous of their colleagues in India. As Harrison notes, most medics in the Indian Service at that time were lower middle class, lower than most British civilians in India, who tended to be professionals. Further, such service was seen as among the least desirable possible appointments by young doctors (Harrison, *Public Health* 15–16, 29–31). Although "tropical" medicine became more central to medical knowledge in the mid-century, and of more interest regarding cholera as medics came closer to theories that accepted a specific disease agent, thus garnering a measure of respect "at home" for these medics' expertise, progress in the two regions' knowledge did not always coincide. When practitioners from India stood on their experience, they could be perceived as high-handed. When James McNabb Cuningham, a medical officer from India, spoke to the Royal Medical and Chirurgical Society in London in 1874, a correspondent to the *British Medical Journal* complained that Cuningham "had been 'arrogant' and 'dismissive of all cholera research in Britain over the last 100 years'" (quoted in Harrison, *Public Health* 110).

18. See Judith Walkowitz.

19. Often this comparison was made explicitly, as in this passage by Mrs. Violet Linley, who compares the epidemics and conditions of the poor in Britain to those in India, point by point: "Almost every malignant disease in this country breaks out among the poor, whose dirty, gossiping propensities spread the evil like wild-fire. Much may be urged in their defence; more ought to be done:—talk of Russian bears, and Indian savages! the poorer classes here are twenty times more uncivilized and worse cared for" (4). The author's attitude toward the poor is hardly what we would term wholly sympathetic, yet she believes that responsibility for aiding them lies with the wealthy; for example, she suggests levying a tax to provide French brandy to the poor. The spirit was considered by her and many others as a specific remedy against cholera and other fevers.

20. See also James Eli Adams, Leonore Davidoff and Catherine Hall, and John Tosh.

21. We might here take note of the way in which drinking was implicated as the typical working-class male abuse of temperance and homeostasis, or bodily control.

22. See especially James Eli Adams, for a full analysis of this dynamic throughout the mid-century.

23. Still, the notion, despite infrequent discussion in the literature, survived; in 1877, Charles Alexander Gordon cautiously observes in *Notes on the Hygiene of Cholera* that "According to some writers the foetus *in utero* has been found dead, its intestines containing the characteristic liquid of cholera evacuations. The presence of the malady in a pregnant woman is considered to tend to abortion" (57). Gordon was an India-based army surgeon and later Surgeon General of the British Army.

24. Lankester was medical officer of St. James's parish. He is best known as a microscopist, but he wrote many works related to sanitation and public health.

25. Still, in 1877, the legend lives on: in a book that gives summaries of medics' findings without commentary or synthesis, Charles Alexander Gordon remarks in a section entitled "IN RELATION TO SEX" that "Cholera has been known to rage violently among, and to be confined to one sex in establishments as at Bristol and elsewhere, containing separate female and male inmates under the same roof, separated only by partitions" (58), but then he continues to give statistics on sex difference that are inconclusive. He also notes that whites seem more liable to it than native Indians (65–67), though that, he cautions, is also inconclusive, and blacks in America seemed to suffer more.

26. Note the problematic relationship of the too-civilized "gentleman" to masculinity.

CHAPTER 7. NARRATING CHOLERA AND NATION

1. Cholera, of course, was a fertile ground for rumors and legends among the middle classes as well as the poor. In her anti-Catholic pamphlet, Mrs. Violet Linley indignantly stated, "We hear of persons taken ill at night, dead in the morning, and buried a few hours afterwards! Was there ever anything so shameful? Verily, a greater encouragement for poisoning and all sorts of crime cannot exist" (7), and indeed, rumours circulated that some had taken advantage of the epidemic to rid themselves of unpleasant spouses, elderly parents, and other incumbrances. The only nondidactic novel I have found that uses the cholera epidemic as a significant element is one by an obscure author, Mrs. Ellen Curd, titled *Ellen Carrington: A Tale of Hull during the Cholera in 1849*. Written in 1875, it reads more like a poorly written sensation novel of the '60s, throwing into the pot every legend of the epidemic that had taken place decades earlier: poisoning under cover of the epidemic to gain an inheritance to pay debts incurred while embezzling; body snatching for the medical school (the apparently dead heroine is discovered to be alive by the medical student about to dissect her); a mad but clairvoyant older female relative who predicts her niece's danger, and so forth. The novel appears to have died quietly on the vine for lack of notice, and so does not figure largely here.

2. All drama with spoken words performed in regular theater venues (not clubs or bars, for example) was submitted to the Lord Chamberlain for approval. References to music hall and burlesque in the press, as we have seen, indicate that the topic was explored there rather cynically, but not much of this material is extant.

3. Kingsley's working-class poet and protagonist, Alton Locke, quotes this as "The Cholera Chaunt," and praises it as one of Mackay's finest poems.

4. Note here that immature constitutions are susceptible to weakening through fright, which affects the sympathetic nervous system.

5. Interestingly, although Bulstrode's disgrace is connected to fiscal irregularities, which lead to the suspicion of murder in a cover-up, Bulstrode is initially susceptible

to disgrace largely because of religious disagreements. (It is notable that the "good" clergyman of the novel is also a naturalist, who trades specimens with Lydgate.) Religious intolerance forms a backdrop to a good deal of the political struggle in the novel.

6. Reform is also tainted in *Middlemarch* by the fiscal selfishness of Brooke, and the opportunity for medical reform is lost when Lydgate compromises himself by association with the fiscal irregularity of Bulstrode—which in turn results from his own fiscal irresponsibility in managing his marriage expenses. The one true reformer in the novel is Ladislaw—the outsider, the disinherited prodigal, victim of Bulstrode. He refuses to be dependent on either Casaubon's or Bulstrode's money, despite the fact that he is ethically entitled to it. Dorothea also renounces her inheritance in choosing to wed Ladislaw in defiance of Casaubon's will. In *Felix Holt*, Esther likewise refuses a tainted inheritance and chooses comparative poverty to be the wife of the radical Felix Holt. Felix himself refuses to be wealthy because he fears he will be compromised by the habits of wealth: "O yes! Your ringed and scented man of the people!—I won't be one of them. Let a man once throttle himself with a satin stock and he'll get new wants and new motives" (91).

CHAPTER 8. KINGSLEY: NATION, GENDER, AND THE BODY

1. Laura Fasick is an exception I take up later. C. J. W. L. Wee has written extensively about Kingsley's racial politics but not about this novel. Please also note that Kingsley's narrator repeatedly refers to Marie as a "quadroon," but he defines her heritage so that she would be understood in this period as an "octoroon," and so I use that term.

2. When Kingsley was confronted with stories of the Indian mutiny, his only solution to the horror with which it filled him was to focus on sanitary reform: "I will forget India in Cholera," he promised (*Life and Works* 73).

3. Laura Fasick points out that Kingsley ignores or has distaste for male slaves (103).

4. Laura Fasick has argued that the Lavington women die because they reject heterosexuality, but, especially in the case of Argemone, this seems unwarranted. The text is explicit that it is the Lavington curse.

5. In contemporary rhetoric, the Crimean epidemic was often linked to the visitation of cholera in Britain, as signs of God's disfavor.

6. Although, as Prickett suggests, Gobineau and others were insistently essentializing race by the early to mid '50s. Joseph Arthur Comte de Gobineau (1816–1882) was a French anthropologist who developing the notion of the Aryan "master race."

7. There are, of course, limits to this monist view of racial hierarchy. The black boy, though he is allowed to play a key role in bringing about the marriage of Stangrave and Marie and averting the duel between Stangrave and Tom, is a static minor character who does not develop and exhibits the most stereoptypical racial traits— dialect speech, dancing, gesturing, grinning (515). Marie, like so many African American heroines of U.S. and British nineteenth-century literature, is light-skinned, and

her ability to transcend racial otherness is based on this. African (and Irish) "wildness" in the *upper* classes is still presented as something to be transcended (though it is at least transcendable), and this otherness, when coded as wildness or barbarism, is less threatening when it is contained in the body of the woman, who herself is defined as appropriately in the position of slave to men. If Marie represents every "nation"—Jewish, Italian, American, African, she also represents a diasporic concept of nationhood that not only defines Jews and Africans, but the British and white Americans as well. The tragic octoroon drama queen can only be domesticated (and anglicized) by men who are willing to fight for her chastity—and containment.

8. Cell theory was current, but Kingsley makes no reference to it, being more interested in analytical chemistry.

9. These figures are according to the World Health Organization's report, *Maternal Mortality in 2000.*

WORKS CITED

"An Account of the Disease Termed Cholera Morbus, from Its First Appearance at Sunderland, to Its Final Departure from Northumberland and Durham, with the Daily Official Reports of Its Destructive Ravages in Newcastle and Gateshead." Newcastle: John Sykes, 1832.

Acland, Henry Wentworth. "An Address to the Inhabitants of St. James's, Westminster on Certain Local Circumstances Affecting the Health of Rich and Poor." London: James Ridgway, 1847.

——— . *Memoir on the Cholera at Oxford in the Year 1854, with Considerations Suggested by the Epidemic.* London: John Churchill; Oxford: J. H. and J. Parker, 1856.

Acton, Lord. "Nationality." *Mapping the Nation.* Ed. Gopal Balakrishnan. New York: Verso, 1996. 17–38.

Adams, James Eli. *Dandies and Desert Saints: Styles of Victorian Masculinity.* Ithaca: Cornell UP, 1995.

"An Affectionate Address to the Inhabitants of Newcastle and Gateshead, and their Vicinity . . . Striking Facts Are Here Adduced." Newcastle-upon-Tyne: Charles Henry Cook, 1832.

"Advice Gratis." *Punch.* 15 (July–Dec. 1848): 207.

Alborn, Timothy L. "A Plague Upon Your Health: Commercial Crisis and Epidemic Disease in Victorian England." *Biology as Society, Society as Biology: Metaphors.* Ed. Sabine Maasen et al. Netherlands: Kluwer Academic P, 1995. 281–310.

Alcock, John. "National Sins and National Calamity: A Sermon Preached in Bethesda Chapel, Dublin, Wed., March 21, 1855." Dublin: Samuel B. Oldham, 1855.

Anderson, Amanda. *The Powers of Distance: Cosmopolitanism and the Cultivation of Detachment.* Princeton: Princeton UP, 2001.

Anderson, Benedict. *Imagined Communities.* [1983] Rev. ed. London: Verso, 1991.

——— . "Introduction." Mapping the Nation. Ed. Gopal Balakrishnan. New York: Verso, 1996. 1–16.

Armstrong, Nancy. *Desire and Domestic Fiction: A Political History of the Novel.* Oxford: Oxford UP, 1987.

Arnold, David. "Cholera and Colonialism in British India." *Past & Present* 113 (1986): 118–51.

———. *Colonizing the Body: State Medicine and Epidemic Disease in Nineteenth-Century India.* Berkeley: U of California P, 1993.

———, Ed. *Imperial Medicine and Indigenous Societies.* Manchester: Manchester UP, 1988.

———. *The Problem of Nature: Environment, Culture, and European Expansion.* London: Blackwell, 1996.

———. "Social Crisis and Epidemic Disease in the Famines of Nineteenth-Century India." *Social History of Medicine* 6.3 (1993): 385–404.

Arnott, Reverend Samuel. "An Address to the Inhabitants of St. Luke's, Berwick Street, Particularly to Those Attending the Church, on the Late Visitation of Cholera." London: William Skeffington, 1854.

Bakhtin, Mikhail. *Rabelais and His World.* Bloomington: Indiana UP, 1984.

Baly, William, M.D., and William W. Gull, M.D. *Reports on the Epidemic Cholera: Drawn Up at the Desire of the Cholera Committee of the Royal College of Physicians.* London: Churchill, 1854.

Banim, Michael. *Chaunt of the Cholera and Songs for Ireland.* London: James Cochrane and Co., 1831.

Barrett Browning, Elizabeth. *Aurora Leigh.* Ed. Margaret Reynolds. New York: W. W. Norton, 1996.

Bartrip, Peter W. J. *Mirror of Medicine: The BMJ 1840–1900.* Oxford: Oxford UP, 1990.

Barua, Dhiman. "History of Cholera." *Cholera.* Dhiman Barua and William B. Greenough. New York: Plenum Medical Book Co., 1992. 1–37.

Barua, Dhiman, and William B. Greenough. *Cholera.* New York: Plenum Medical Book Co., 1992.

Best, Geoffrey. *Honour Among Men and Nations: Transformations of an Idea.* Toronto: U of Toronto P, 1981.

Bewell, Alan. *Romanticism and Colonial Disease.* Baltimore: Johns Hopkins UP, 1999.

Bhabha, Homi K. "DissemiNation: Time, Narrative, and the Margins of the Modern Nation." *Nation and Narration.* Ed. Homi K. Bhabha. London and New York: Routledge, 1990. 291–322.

Bichat, Xavier. "Physiological Researches on Life and Death." *Significant Contributions to the History of Psychology, 1750–1920.* Vol. 2. Ed. Daniel N. Robinson. Washington, D.C.: University Publications of America, 1978.

Bickersteth, Edward. "Parochial and Congregational Fasting, on Occasion of the Cholera in 1849." London: Seeleys, 1849.

Billing, Archibald, M.D. *First Principles of Medicine.* London: Thomas and George Underwood, 1831.

———. *First Principles of Medicine.* 5th ed. London: S. Highley, 1849.

Bland, Philip. "God's Warning, and the People's Duty: A Sermon Preached at St. Mary's Church, Rotherhithe, on Sunday morning, July 15, 1849, during the Severe Visitation of the Cholera." London: Wertheim and Macintosh, 1849.

Bourdelais, Patrice. *Une peur bleue: histoire du choléra en France 1832–1854.* Paris: Payot, 1987.

Bourdieu, Pierre. *Distinction: A Social Critique of the Judgement of Taste.* Trans. Richard Nice. Cambridge, Mass.: Harvard UP, 1984.

Braithwaite, William. "God's Judgements." London: Joseph Masters, 1849.

Brantlinger, Patrick. *Fictions of State: Culture and Credit in Britain, 1694–1994.* Ithaca: Cornell UP, 1996.

———. *Rule of Darkness: British Literature and Imperialism, 1830–1914.* Ithaca: Cornell UP, 1988.

———. *The Spirit of Reform: British Literature and Politics, 1832–1867.* Cambridge, Mass.: Harvard UP, 1977.

Bristowe, John Syer, M.D., F.R.C.P. *The Theory and Practice of Medicine.* 3rd ed. London: Smith, Elder, & Co., 1880.

Broadsheet. "Cholera Humbug: The Arrival and Departure of the Cholera Morbus." J.V. Quick, printer: Clerkenwell, 1832.

Broadsheet. "Cholera Morbus!" T. Hodge, Sutherland, printer: 10 Nov., 1381 [*sic*—actually 1831].

Broadsheet. "A New Song on the Cholera Morbus." Quarto Broadsheet: London Guildhall, Ephemera Collection. Wheeler, printer: 1831 (?).

Broadsheet. Place collection. Jocelyne, printer: Braintree, 22 Mar., 1847.

Broadsheet. "There Is No Such Disorder Now Existing in Our Town." Guildhall Collection. T. Kidderminster. Pennell, printer: 2 October, 1832.

Brose, Olive J. *Church and Parliament: The Reshaping of the Church of England, 1828–1860.* London and Stanford: Stanford UP, 1959.

Buchanan, Robert. "The Waste Places of Our Great Cities: Or, the Voice of God in the Cholera. With Remarks on the Recent Letter upon That Subject of the Right Hon. Lord Palmerston." Third thousand. Glasgow: Blackie and Son, 1853.

Buckland, William. "A Sermon Preached in Westminster Abbey, on the 15th Day of November, 1849, Being the Day of Thanksgiving to God for the Removal of the Cholera." London: John Murray, 1849.

Burton, Antoinette. *Burdens of History: British Feminists, Indian Women, and Imperial Culture, 1865–1915.* Chapel Hill: U of North Carolina P, 1994.

By the Author of "A Letter to Everybody." "Why Are You Afraid of the Cholera? . . . (with Medical Directions)." London: no publisher, 1832.

Calthrop, Gordon. "If the Cholera Comes, How Are We to Interpret It: A Sermon Preached at St. Augustine's Church, Highbury New Park, London 1865." London: Wm. Hunt and Co., 1865.

Carleton, Mrs. "Enquiry into the Nature of the Choleraic Influence, Its Origin and Its Course, to Which Is Added a Collection of the Most Effectual Remedies for the Cholera Adopted in Various Countries and a Plan of Treatment by the Author." London: H. Bailliere, 1866.

Chadwick, Edwin. *Report on the Labouring Population of Great Britain.* London: 1842.

Chapman, John, M.D. *Diarrhoea and Cholera: Their Nature, Origin and Treatment, through the Agency of the Nervous System.* 2nd ed. enlarged. London: Trubner and Co., 1866.

Chapman, Raymond. "Charles Kingsley and the Lavington Curse." *Notes and Queries.* 18 (1971): 91.

"Cholera." *Times.* 21 Dec. 1854: 7.

"The Cholera and Its Effects, as Connected with the Operations of the London City Mission." *London City Mission Magazine.* 14 (October 1849): 199–226.

"The Cholera." *Press and St. James Chronicle.* 11 Aug. 1866: 508.

"Cholera in the City." *City Press.* 1 Sept. 1866: 3.

"Cholera in Whitechapel." *Times.* 20 Dec. 1848: no page number.

Clark, J. C. D. *English Society: 1688–1832.* Cambridge: Cambridge UP, 1985.

Clinical Lectures. Manuscripts in the archive of the Royal College of Physicians.

Coleman, B. I. *The Church of England in the Mid-Nineteenth Century: A Social Geography.* London: The Historical Association, 1980.

Coles, Nicholas. "Sinners in the Hands of an Angry Utilitarian." *Bulletin of Research in the Humanities* 86 (1983–1985): 153–88.

Colley, Linda. *Britons: Forging the Nation, 1707–1837.* New Haven: Yale UP, 1992.

Crosby, Alfred. *Ecological Imperialism: The Biological Expansion of Europe, 900–1900.* Cambridge: Cambridge UP, 1993.

Cullen, William. *Synopsis Nosologicae Medicae.* Edinburgh: William Creech, 1785

Curd, Mrs. *Ellen Carrington: A Tale of Hull during the Cholera in 1849.* Hull: Thornton and Patterson, 1875.

Davidoff, Leonore, and Catherine Hall. *Family Fortunes: Men and Women of the English Middle Class 1780–1850.* London: Routledge, 1992.

Davies, John. "The Responsibility Entailed by the Past: A Sermon Preached at St. Mary's Church, Gateshead on the Public Thanksgiving Day, after the Removal of the Cholera, Thursday, October 27, 1853." London: Seeleys, 1853.

Delaporte, François. *Disease and Civilization: The Cholera in Paris, 1832.* Trans. Arthur Goldhammer; foreword by Paul Rabinow. Cambridge: MIT P, 1986.

Dickens, Charles. *Bleak House*. Oxford: Oxford UP, 1998.

"Didymus." "The Public Fast." *Wesleyan Methodist Magazine* [London]. LV (April 1832): 257–64.

———. "Weekly Intercession Meeting." *Wesleyan Methodist Magazine* [London]. LIV (December 1831): 12–15.

Digby, Anne. *Making a Medical Living: Doctors and Patients in the English Market for Medicine, 1720–1911*. Cambridge: Cambridge UP, 1994.

Disraeli, Benjamin. *Sybil, or The Two Nations*. Oxford: Oxford UP, 1981.

Donzelot, Jacques. *The Policing of Families*. With a foreword by Gilles Deleuze; translated from the French by Robert Hurley. New York: Pantheon Books, 1979.

Durbach, Nadja. *Bodily Matters: The Anti-Vaccination Movement in England, 1853–1907*. Durham and London: Duke UP, 2005.

Durey, Michael. *The Return of the Plague: British Society and the Cholera, 1831–2*. Dublin: Gill and Macmillan Humanities P, 1979.

Editors. *Lancet* 1 (Nov. 24, 1832): 270.

Edson, Cyrus. "The Microbe as Social Leveller." *The North American Review* 161 (1895): 421–26.

Elias, Norbert. *The Civilizing Process*. New York: Pantheon Books, 1982.

Eliot, George. *Daniel Deronda*. Oxford: Oxford UP, 1998.

———. *Felix Holt, The Radical*. Toronto: Broadview, 2000.

———. *Middlemarch*. New York: Bantam, 1992.

———. *Mill on the Floss*. New York: W. W. Norton and Co., 1994.

Elliott, Henry Venn. "Two Sermons on the Hundred and First and Sixty-Second Psalms as Applicable to the Harvest, the Cholera, and the War." London: T. Hatcherd, 1854.

Evans, Richard J. *Death in Hamburg: Society and Politics in the Cholera Years, 1830–1910*. Oxford: Clarendon P, 1987.

———. "Epidemics and Revolutions: Cholera in Nineteenth-Century Europe." *Past and Present* 120 (1988): 123–46.

Eyler, John M. *Victorian Social Medicine: The Ideas and Methods of William Farr*. Baltimore: Johns Hopkins UP, 1979.

Farr, William. "Influence of Elevation on Fatality of Cholera." *Journal of the Royal Statistical Society* 15 (1852): 155–83.

———. *Vital Statistics: A Memorial Volume of Selections from the Reports and Writings of William Farr*. Introduction by Mervyn Susser and Abraham Adelstein. Metuchen, N.J.: Scarecrow Press, 1975.

Fasick, Laura. "Charles Kingsley's Scientific Treatment of Gender." *Muscular Christianity: Embodying the Victorian Age*. Ed. Donald Hall. Cambridge: Cambridge UP, 1994. 91–113.

Finn, Margot C. *After Chartism: Class and Nation in English Radical Politics, 1848–1874.* Cambridge: Cambridge UP, 1993.

Flint, Kate. *The Woman Reader, 1837–1914.* Oxford: Oxford UP, 1993.

Foucault, Michel. *The Birth of the Clinic.* [1963]. New York: Pantheon, 1973.

———. "Governmentality." *The Foucault Effect: Studies in Governmentality.* Ed. Graham Burchell, Colin Gordon, and Peter Miller. Chicago: U of Chicago P, 1991.

———. *The Order of Things.* [1966]. New York: Pantheon, 1970.

Fowler, Robert, M.D. "Cholera in the City." *City Press.* 1 Sept. 1866: 3.

Fox, Oscar. Letter. Dated Friday, 14 Sept. 1849. Guildhall Records Office.

Gallagher, Catherine. *The Body Economic: Life, Death, and Sensation in Political Economy and the Victorian Novel.* Princeton: Princeton UP, 2005.

———. "The Body versus the Social Body in the Works of Thomas Malthus and Henry Mayhew." *Representations* XIV (1986): 83–106.

———. *The Industrial Reformation of English Fiction: Social Discourse and Narrative Form 1832–1867.* Chicago: U of Chicago P, 1985.

Gaselee, Charles, and Alexander Tweedie. *A Practical Treatise on the Cholera, as It Has Appeared in Various Parts of the Metropolis.* London: [publisher unreadable], 1832.

Gaulter, Henry, M.D. *The Origin and Progress of the Malignant Cholera in Manchester.* London: Longman, and Manchester: Harison and Crosfield, 1833.

Gellner, Ernest. *Nations and Nationalism.* Ithaca: Cornell UP, 1983.

General Board of Health, Medical Council. *Appendix to Report of the Committee for Scientific Inquiries in Relation to the Cholera Epidemic of 1854.* London: Eyre and Spottiswoode, 1855.

Giddens, Anthony. *The Constitution of Society: Outline of the Theory of Structuration.* Berkeley: U of California P, 1984.

Gilbert, Pamela K. *The Citizen's Body: Desire, Health and the Social in Victorian England.* Columbus: Ohio State University Press, 2007.

———. *Mapping the Victorian Social Body.* Albany: State U of New York P, 2004.

Godwin, George. *Town Swamps and Social Bridges: The Sequel to a Glance at the Homes of the Thousands.* London: Routledge, Warnes and Routledge, 1859.

Goodeve, Edward. "Epidemic Cholera." *A System of Medicine.* Ed. J. Russell Reynolds, M.D., F.R.C.P. London: Macmillan, 1866. 26–188.

Goodlad, Lauren. *Victorian Literature and the Victorian State: Character and Governance in a Liberal Society.* Baltimore: Johns Hopkins UP, 2003.

Gordon, Sir Charles Alexander, K.C.B. *Notes on the Hygiene of Cholera, for Ready Reference.* London: 1877. Also published in Madras: Gantz Brothers; Calcutta and Bombay, Spink and Co., 1877.

Grainger, R. D. *Appendix B to The Report of the General Board of Health on the Epidemic Cholera of 1848–1849*. London: Printed by W. Clowes and Sons, for Her Majesty's Stationery Office, 1850.

———. Letter. 13 Sept. 1849. Guildhall Collection of Letters to the Metropolitan Commissioners of Sewers.

Granshaw, Lindsay. "Knowledge of Bodies or Bodies of Knowledge? Surgeons, Anatomists and Rectal Surgery, 1830–1985 [*sic*]." *Medical Theory, Surgical Practice*. Ed. Christopher Lawrence. London: Routledge, 1992. 232–62.

Gregory, George, M.D., L.R.C.P. *Elements of the Theory and Practice of Medicine: Designed for the Use of Students and Junior Practitioners*. 4th ed. London: Baldwin and Craddock, 1835.

———. *Elements of the Theory and Practice of Medicine: Designed for the Use of Students and Junior Practitioners* . 6th ed. London: Henry Renshaw, 1846.

Grove, John, M.D. "On Epidemic Cholera and Diarrhoea: Their Prevention and Treatment by Sulphur." 3rd ed. London: Robert Hardwick, 1865.

Hacking, Ian. *The Taming of Chance*. Cambridge: Cambridge UP, 1990.

Hall, Donald. "On the Making and Unmaking of Monsters: Christian Socialism, Muscular Christianity, and the Metaphorization of Class Conflict." *Muscular Christianity: Embodying the Victorian Age*. Ed. Donald Hall. Cambridge: Cambridge UP, 1994. 45–65.

Haley, Bruce. *The Healthy Body and Victorian Culture*. Cambridge, Mass.: Harvard UP, 1978.

Hamlin, Christopher. *Public Health and Social Justice in the Age of Chadwick: Britain, 1800–1854*. Cambridge: Cambridge UP, 1998.

———. *A Science of Impurity: Water Analysis in Nineteenth-Century Britain*. Bristol: Adam Hilger, 1990.

Harrison, Mark. *Climates and Constitutions*. New Delhi: Oxford UP, 1999.

———. *Public Health in British India: Anglo-Indian Preventive Medicine, 1859–1914*. Cambridge: Cambridge UP, 1994.

Haywood, William. Letter Books of William Haywood, Commissioners of Sewers. 11 Sept. 1849. Guildhall Collection of Letters to the Metropolitan Commissioners of Sewers.

"The Health of Shoreditch." *Shoreditch Observer*. 8 Sept. 1866: 3.

Hetherington, Henry. *The Poor Man's Guardian* 1:1 (1832): 274.

Hobsbawm, Eric. *Nations and Nationalism since 1788*. Cambridge: Cambridge UP, 1990.

———, and Terence Ranger, Eds. *The Invention of Tradition*. Cambridge: Cambridge UP, 1983.

Holmes, Reginald. *That Alarming Malady*. Ely Local History Series. (Copyright Reg. Holmes, 1974. Printed by the Ely Local History Publication Board).

Huelin, G. "The Church's Response to the Cholera Outbreak of 1866." *Studies in Church History* 6: 137–48.

Hughes, Thomas Snead. "A Sermon [on Psalm lxxv. 7] Preached October 7, 1857, the Day of General Humiliation, and Prayer . . . for the Restoration of Tranquillity in India." London: no publisher, 1857.

Hume, John Chandler. "Colonialism and Sanitary Medicine: The Development of Preventive Health Policy in the Punjab, 1860 to 1900." *Modern Asian Studies* 28 (1986): 703–24.

Jarman, Rev. D. F. (David Fenton). "The Cholera, Its True Cause and Its Only Cure, Set Forth in Two Discourses." London: W. F. Crofts, [1849?].

Johnson, George, M.D. "On Cholera and Choleraic Diarrhoea; Their Nature, Cause and Treatment: Two Lectures, Delivered at The Church Missionary College, Islington." London: John Churchill and Sons, 1870.

Joyce, Patrick. *Democratic Subjects: The Self and the Social in Nineteenth-Century England*. Cambridge: Cambridge UP, 1994.

Kay-Shuttleworth, James Phillips. *The Moral and Physical Condition of the Working Classes Employed in the Cotton Manufacture in Manchester*. London: James Ridgway, 1832.

Keble, John. *Sermons, Academical and Occasional*. London: no publisher, 1848.

Kell, Edmund. "What Patriotism, Justice, and Christianity Demand for India: A sermon [on Matt. vii. 12]." London, Southampton: E. T. Whitfield, 1857.

Kilgour, Maggie. *From Communion to Cannibalism: An Anatomy of Metaphors of Incorporation*. Princeton: Princeton UP, 1990.

Kingsley, Charles. *Cheap Clothes and Nasty: By Parson Lot*. London: W. Pickering, 1850.

———. *Letters and Memories, Edited by His Wife*. New York: Co-operative Publication Society, 1899.

———. *The Life and Works of Charles Kingsley*. 19 vols. London: Macmillan and Co., Limited; New York: Macmillan, 1901–1903.

———. *Novels, Poems and Letters of Charles Kingsley*. 1–2 *Alton Locke*. Bideford Edition. New York: Co-operative Publication Society [1898–1899].

———. *Novels, Poems and Letters of Charles Kingsley*. 5–6 *Hereward the Wake*. Bideford Edition. New York: Co-operative Publication Society [1898–1899].

———. *Novels, Poems and Letters of Charles Kingsley*. 7–8 *Hypatia*. Bideford Edition. New York: Co-operative Publication Society [1898–1899].

———. *Two Years Ago*. New York: Macmillan, 1877.

———. *The Water-Babies*. Oxford: Oxford UP, 1995.

———. *Westward Ho!* New York: Scribner, 1920.

———. *Yeast: A Problem*. New York, Macmillan, 1902.

Klein, Ira. "Cholera, Dysentery and Development in Eastern India 1871–1921." *Journal of Indian History* Golden Jubilee Volume (1973): 805–20.

———. "Death in India, 1871–1921." *Journal of Asian Studies* 32.4 (1973): 639–59.

———. "Imperialism, Ecology and Disease: Cholera in India, 1850–1950." *Indian Economic and Social History Review* 31.4 (1994): 491–518.

Kristeva, Julia. *Desire in Language: A Semiotic Approach to Literature and Art*. Trans. Thomas Gora, Alice Jardine, and Leon S. Roudiez. Ed. Leon S. Roudiez. New York: Columbia UP, 1980.

Kudlick, Catherine. *Cholera in Post-Revolutionary Paris: A Cultural History*. Berkeley: U of California P, 1996.

Kushner, Tony. *Angels in America: A Gay Fantasia on National Themes*. New York: Theater Communications Group, 2003.

Ladies' Sanitary Association. "The Use of Pure Water." 14th ed. Sixty-eight thousand. London: Jarrold and Sons, 2d. [not dated, probably mid to late 1860s].

———. "Village Work." London: S. W. Partridge, [1867?].

The *Lancet*. 2. 1831–1832.

Lane, Christopher. *The Ruling Passion: British Colonial Allegory and the Paradox of Homosexual Desire*. Durham: Duke UP, 1995.

Lankester, Edwin, M.D. *Cholera: What Is It and How to Prevent It*. London: George Routledge and Sons, 1866.

Laqueur, Thomas Walter. *Making Sex: Body and Gender from the Greeks to Freud*. Cambridge, Mass.: Harvard UP, 1990.

Lawrence, Christopher. "Democratic, Divine and Heroic: The History and Historiography of Surgery." *Medical Theory, Surgical Practice*. Ed. Christopher Lawrence. London: Routledge, 1992. 1–47.

Lawrence, Susan C. *Charitable Knowledge: Hospital Pupils and Practitioners in Eighteenth-Century London*. Cambridge: Cambridge UP, 1996.

"The Laws of Cholera." Rpt. from the *Times*, with an introduction and supplementary matter. London: Charles Knight, [1853?].

Lawson, Emily. *Through Tumult and Pestilence*. London: SPCK, 1886.

Lewis, Jane. "Presidential Address: Family Provision of Health and Welfare in the Mixed Economy of Care in the late Nineteenth and Twentieth Centuries." *Social History of Medicine* 8.1 (April 1995): 1–16.

Lewis, Roy, and Angus Maude. *Professional People in England*. Cambridge, Mass.: Harvard UP, 1953.

Levine, Philippa. *Prostitution, Race, and Politics: Policing Venereal Disease in the British Empire*. New York: Routledge, 2003.

Linley, Mrs. Violet. "Cholera: A Word for the Future." London: Thomas Harrison, 1854.

London Cholera Hospital Casebooks, 1832. Manuscripts in the archive of the Royal College of Physicians. 1832.

Loudon, Irvine. *Medical Care and the General Practitioner 1750–1850.* Oxford: Clarendon P, 1986.

Lyon, Eileen Groth. *Politicians in the Pulpit: Christian Radicalism in Britain from the Fall of the Bastille to the Disintegration of Chartism.* Aldershot, Hants: Ashgate, 1999.

MacPherson, John, M.D. *Cholera in Its Home, with a Sketch of the Pathology and Treatment of the Disease.* London: John Churchill and Sons, 1866.

Mackay, Charles. "The Mowers: An Anticipation of the Cholera, 1848." http://www.firstscience.com/SITE/poemsmackay. Accessed 23 May 2004.

Mann, Thomas. *Death in Venice and Seven Other Stories by Thomas Mann.* Trans. H. T. Lowe-Porter. New York: Vintage, 1930.

"Mansion House Cholera Relief Committee." *City Press.* 15 Sept. 1866: 3.

Marsh, Catherine. "Death and Life: A Record of the Cholera Wards in the London Hospital." London: James Nisbet, 1866.

Marshall, T. H., with Tom Bottomore. *Citizenship and Social Class.* London: Pluto P, 1992.

Martineau, Harriet. *Deerbrook: A Novel.* New York: The Dial Press, Doubleday and Co., 1984.

M'Carthy, J. M. and Mrs. Dove. "Abstract of Notes of the Cholera Cases under the care of Dr. A. Clark, w/Remarks." Clinical Lectures and Reports. Vol. 3 (1866). East London Hospital Archive.

McClintock, Anne. *Imperial Leather: Race, Gender, and Sexuality in the Colonial Contest.* New York: Routledge, 1995.

McCormack, Kathleen. *George Eliot and Intoxication: Dangerous Drugs for the Condition of England.* London: Macmillan, 2000.

McGrew, Roderick E. *Russia and the Cholera, 1823–1832.* Madison: U of Wisconsin P, 1965.

Menninghaus, Winfried. *Disgust: The Theory and History of a Strong Sensation.* Trans. Howard Eiland and Joel Golb. Albany: State U of New York P, 2003.

"Metropolitan Confusions." *City Press.* Sat., 14 July 1866: 4.

Metz, Nancy Aycock. "Discovering a World of Suffering: Fiction and the Rhetoric of Sanitary Reform—1840–1860," *Nineteenth-Century Contexts* 15.1 (1991): 65–81.

M'Neile, Hugh. "Confession without Amendment, or Dissembling with God: A Sermon Suggested by the Special Prayer against the Cattle Plague and Cholera: Preached in Chester Cathedral and Published by Request." London: Hatchard and Co.; Liverpool: Edward Howell, 1866.

Morris, R. J. *Cholera 1832: The Social Response to an Epidemic.* London: Croom Helm, 1976.

Mort, Frank. *Dangerous Sexualities: Medico-Moral Politics in England since 1830.* London and New York: Routledge and Kegan Paul, 1987.

"National Improvement." *Lancet* 1 (1831–1832): 2.

Nicholls, Phillip A. *Homeopathy and the Medical Profession.* London: Croom Helm, 1988.

O'Connor, Erin. *Raw Material: Producing Pathology in Victorian Culture.* Durham: Duke UP, 2000.

Orton, Reginald. *An Essay on the Epidemic Cholera of India. 2nd ed., with a Supplement.* Burgess and Hill: London, 1831.

Parkin, John. *The Antidotal Treatment of the Epidemic Cholera.* London: Sampson, Low, Marston and Co., 1836.

———. *The Antidotal Treatment of the Epidemic Cholera.* 2nd edition. London: Sampson, Low, Marston and Co., 1848.

———. *The Antidotal Treatment of the Epidemic Cholera.* 3rd ed. London: Sampson, Low, Marston and Co., 1866. (material cited is from this edition)

Parliamentary Papers. Irish University Press series of British Parliamentary Papers. 1000-Volume Series 1801–1899. Shannon: Irish University Press.

Pelling, Margaret. *Cholera, Fever, and English Medicine, 1825–1865.* Oxford: Oxford UP, 1978.

Perkin, Harold. *The Origins of Modern English Society 1780–1880.* London: Routledge & K. Paul; Toronto: U of Toronto P, 1969.

Peterson, Jeanne. *The Medical Profession in Mid-Victorian London.* Berkeley: U of California P, 1978.

Pickstone, John V. "Ferriar's Fever to Kay's Cholera: Disease and Social Structure in Cottonopolis." *History of Science* 22.4 (1984): 401–19.

Place Collection. [a collection of clippings and other printed items held in the British Library]. *Times.* 18 Jan. 1848. [no title].

"Plunder of Cholera Patients." *St. James's Chronicle.* 19 July 1849.

Poor Man's Guardian. 1832.

Poovey, Mary. *Making a Social Body: British Cultural Formation, 1830–1864.* Chicago: U of Chicago P, 1995.

Porter, Rev. J. Leech. "National Christianity for India, or National Acts and National Duties Viewed in Connection to the Sepoy Mutinies." London: Wertheim and Macintosh, 1857.

Power, Sir Alfred. K.C.B. *Sanitary Rhymes: Personal Precautions against Cholera, and All Kinds of Fever, etc.* London: T. Richards, 1871.

Prashad, Vijay. "Native Dirt/Imperial Ordure: The Cholera of 1832 and the Morbid Resolutions of Modernity." *Journal of Historical Sociology* 7.3 (1994): 243–60.

"Precautions against Cholera." *Times.* Wed., 25 July 1866: no page number.

Prickett, Stephen. "Purging Christianity of Its Semitic Origins: Kingsley, Arnold and the Bible." *Rethinking Victorian Culture.* Ed. Juliet John and Alice Jenkins. Basingstoke: Macmillan, 2000. 63–79.

"A Protest against the Prayer for the Cholera, Lately Issued and Still in Use, as Being both Irreligious and Unorthodox." London: William Freeman, 1866.

"The Public Health Bill." *Times.* Sat., 28 July 1866: 7–8.

Ramasubban, Radhika. "Imperial Health in British India: 1857–1900." *Disease, Medicine and Empire.* Ed. Roy MacLeod and Milton Lewis. London: Routledge, 1988. 38–60.

Rees, George, M.D. *Lectures, Delivered at the Mechanics Institute, 19th Dec. 1831, and 13th Feb. 1832, on Carbon, Oxygen and Vitality, . . . with Remarks on Asiatic Cholera.* London: Highly, Fleet Street and Hookham, Bond Street, 1832.

"Report on the Cases Treated in the Wapping District Cholera Hospital" (by Dr. W.B. Woodman, and Mr. N. Hickford, in casebooks, pp. 471–84.) In archive of East London Hospital.

Report on the Cholera Outbreak in the Parish of St. James, Westminster, During the Autumn of 1854: Presented to the Vestry by The Cholera Inquiry Committee, July 1855. London: J. Churchill, 1855.

Report of the Committee for Scientific Inquiries: Irish University Press Series of British Parliamentary Papers: Reports on the Epidemics of 1854 and 1866 and Other Reports on Cholera with Appendices: Health, Infectious Diseases 3. Shannon, Ireland: Irish UP, 1970. 5–67.

Report of the General Board of Health on the Epidemic Cholera of 1848–1849. London: Printed by W. Clowes and Sons, for Her Majesty's Stationery Office, 1850.

Report to the International Sanitary Conference, of a Commission from that Body on the Origin, Endemicity, Transmissability and Propagation of Asiatic Cholera. Trans. Samuel L. Abot, M.D. Boston: Alfred Mudge and Sons, 1867.

"Retrospective of Public Affairs." *Wesleyan Methodist Magazine* [London]. LV (Feb. 1832): 148–51.

Reynolds, James Russell, M.D., F.R.C.P., ed. *A System of Medicine.* 5 vols. London: Macmillan, 1866.

———, ed. *A System of Medicine.* 3rd ed. 5 vols. London: Macmillan, 1876.

Richards, Thomas. *The Commodity Culture of Victorian Britain: Advertising and Spectacle, 1851–1914.* Stanford: Stanford UP, 1990.

———. *The Imperial Archive: Knowledge and the Fantasy of Empire.* London: Verso, 1993.

Richardson, Ruth. *Death, Dissection and the Destitute.* London: Routledge, 1987.

Robinson, Archibald. "Treatment of the Malignant Cholera on Board the Cumberland Convict Hulk." *Lancet* 2 (1831–1832): 557–59.

Rodger, Richard. *Housing in Urban Britain 1780–1914: Class Capitalism and Construction.* London: Macmillan, 1989.

Rose, Nikolas S. *Powers of Freedom: Reframing Political Thought.* Cambridge: Cambridge UP, 1999.

Rosenberg, Charles. *Explaining Epidemics and Other Studies in the History of Medicine.* Cambridge: Cambridge UP, 1992.

Rothfield, Lawrence. *Vital Signs: Medical Realism in Nineteenth-Century Fiction.* Princeton: Princeton UP, 1992.

Sanderson, William. "Suggestions in Reference to the Present Cholera Epidemic, for the Purification of the Water Supply and the Reclamation of East London, with Remarks on the Origin of the Cholera Poison." London: William Macintosh, 1866.

Sansom, Arthur Ernest. *The Arrest and Prevention of Cholera: Being a Guide to the Antiseptic Treatment with New Observations on Causation.* London: John Churchill and Sons, 1866.

SDUK (Society for the Diffusion of Useful Knowledge). *The Working Man's Companion: The Physician 1. The Cholera.* London: Charles Knight, 1832.

Sedgwick, William, MRCS. *On the Nature of Cholera as a Guide to Treatment.* 2nd ed. London: Walton and Maberly, 1866.

Sensus Communis (Psued.) "The Cholera: No Judgement! The Efficacy, Philosophy and Practical Tendency of the Prayer by the Archbishop of Canterbury Ordered to Be Used during the Prevalence of Cholera, Examined in a Letter Addressed to the Right Honorable the Earl of Carlisle, Chief Commissioner of Woods and Forests, President of the Board of Public Heath, etc., etc." London: Aylott and Jones, 1849.

Shapter, Thomas. *The Cholera in Exeter in 1832.* Republished, Wakefield and London: S. R. Republishers Ltd., 1971.

Shlomowitz, Ralph, and Lance Brennan. "Mortality and Migrant Labour *en route* to Assam, 1863–1924." *Indian Economic and Social History Review* 27.3 (1990): 313–30.

Simon, John. Letter Addressed to the London Committee on Health, 2 Oct. 1849. Guildhall Collection of Letters to the Metropolitan Commissioners of Sewers.

Sinha, Mrinalini. *The "Manly Englishman" and the "Effeminate Bengali" in the Late Nineteenth Century.* Manchester: Manchester UP; New York: St. Martin's Press, 1995.

Smiles, Samuel. *Self-Help: With Illustrations of Character and Good Conduct.* London: [John] Murray, 1859.

Snow, John. *On the Mode of Communication of Cholera.* 2nd ed., much enlarged. London: John Churchill, 1855.

———. "On the Pathology and Mode of Communication of Cholera." Tract reprinted from the *London Medical Gazette* 44. London: no publisher, 1849.

———. *Snow on Cholera: Being a Reprint of Two Papers by John Snow, M.D., Together with a Biographical Memoir by B. W. Richardson, M.D., and an Introduction by Wade Hampton Frost, M.D.* New York: The Commonwealth Fund. London and Oxford: Oxford UP, 1936.

Spencer, Herbert. Essay. *Leader.* 20 March 1852. http://www.clarehall.cam.ac.uk/userpages/djhc2/contbib/spencer.htm. Accessed 10 November 2000.

———. *Social Statics.* New York: Robert Schalkenbach Foundation, 1954.

"St. Olave's District Board of Works." [minutes of meeting] *South London Press.* 25 Aug. 1866: 4.

"Suggestions for the Prevention of the Cholera." *City Press.* 11 Aug. 1866.

Sugden, Samuel. "Letter from Tipton." Religious Intelligences section. *The Wesleyan Methodist Magazine* (Nov. 1832): 819–20.

Suleri, Sara. *The Rhetoric of English India.* Chicago: U of Chicago P, 1992.

"Supplement to the Report of the Committee for Scientific Inquiries." *Irish University Press Series of British Parliamentary Papers: Reports on the Epidemics of 1854 and 1866 and Other Reports on Cholera with Appendices: Health, Infectious Diseases 3.* Shannon, Ireland: Irish UP, 1970. 81–143.

Sussman, Herbert L. *Victorian Masculinities: Manhood and Masculine Poetics in Early Victorian Literature and Art.* Cambridge: Cambridge UP, 1995.

Tanner, Thomas Hawkes. *The Practice of Medicine.* 2 vols. 6th ed. London: Henry Renshaw, 1869.

Taylor, James A. "The Cholera: Or, God's Voice in the Pestilence, a Sermon." London: no publisher, 1832.

Tosh, John. *A Man's Place: Masculinity and the Middle-Class Home in Victorian England.* New Haven: Yale UP, 1999.

"Two Sermons on the Hundred and First and Sixty-Second Psalms as Applicable to the Harvest, the Cholera, and the War." London: T. Hatcherd, 1854.

"Untitled." *Times.* 24 Feb. 1848.

Verdery, Katherine. "Whither 'Nation' and 'Nationalism'?" *Mapping the Nation.* Ed. Gopal Balakrishnan. Intro. Benedict Anderson. New York: Verso, 1996. 226–34.

Wakley, Thomas. "Untitled." *Lancet* 2 (1831–1832): 218–21.

Walby, Sylvia. "Woman and Nation." *Mapping the Nation.* Ed. Gopal Balakrishnan, Intro. Benedict Anderson. London: Verso, 1996. 235–54.

Walkowitz, Judith R. *City of Dreadful Delight: Narratives of Sexual Danger in Late Victorian London.* Chicago: U of Chicago P, 1992.

Watts, Sheldon J. *Epidemics and History: Disease, Power, and Imperialism.* New Haven: Yale UP, 1997.

Wee, C. J. W. L. "Christian Manliness and National Identity: The Problematic Construction of a Racially 'Pure' Nation." *Muscular Christianity: Embodying the Victorian Age.* Ed. Donald Hall. Cambridge: Cambridge UP, 1994. 66–88.

"West London Union" section of "The Cholera." *City Press*. 11 Aug. 1866: 6.

[Whitehead, Henry.] "The Cholera in Berwick St." By the Curate of St. Luke's. 2nd ed. London: Hope and Co., 1854.

Whittaker, D. K. "The Cholera Conference." *London Quarterly Review* 27 (Jan. 1867): 16–29.

Wilkinson, James John Garth. *War, Cholera, and the Ministry of Health: An Appeal to Sir Benjamin Hall and the British People.* London: no publisher, 1854.

Williams, Raymond. *The Country and the City.* New York: Oxford UP, 1973.

Winslow, Forbes. "The Cholera, Considered Psychologically." London: J. Churchill, 1849.

Witz, Anne. *Professions and Patriarchy.* London: Routledge, 1992.

Woodman, Dr. W. B., and Mr. N. Hickford. "Report on the Cases Treated in the Wapping District Cholera Hospital." Casebooks held in the Archive of London Hospital. 471–84.

World Health Organization. *Maternal Mortality in 2000.* http://www.who.int/reproductive-health/publications/maternal_mortality_2000/index.html. Accessed 11 April 2006.

Wright, Thomas Giordani. *Cholera in the Asylum: Reports on the Origin and Progress of Pestilential Cholera in the West-Yorkshire Lunatic Asylum, during the Autumn of 1849.* London, Wakefield: Longmans & Co. [printed], 1850.

Yonge, Charlotte Mary. *The Heir of Redclyffe.* Illus. Kate Greenaway. New York: Macmillan, 1900.

——— . *The Three Brides.* 2 vols. London: Macmillan, 1876.

Žižek, Slavoj. *The Sublime Object of Ideology.* London: Verso, 1989.

INDEX